Rowan's
PRIMER *of* **EEG**

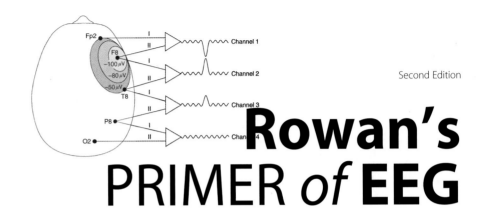

Second Edition

Rowan's PRIMER *of* EEG

LARA V MARCUSE MD
Assistant Professor Neurology and
Co-Director of the Mount Sinai Epilepsy Center,
The Icahn School of Medicine at Mount Sinai,
New York, USA

MADELINE C FIELDS MD
Assistant Professor Neurology and
Co-Director of the Mount Sinai Epilepsy Center,
The Icahn School of Medicine at Mount Sinai,
New York, USA

JIYEOUN (JENNA) YOO MD
Assistant Professor Neurology,
The Mount Sinai Epilepsy Center,
The Icahn School of Medicine at Mount Sinai,
New York, USA

Foreword
Jacqueline A French MD
Professor of Neurology,
New York University Comprehensive Epilepsy Center,
Chief Scientific Officer, Epilepsy Foundation,
New York, USA

For additional online content visit expertconsult.com

ELSEVIER

Edinburgh   London   New York   Oxford   Philadelphia   St Louis   Sydney   Toronto 2016

ELSEVIER

First edition 2003
Second edition 2016

Notices
Knowledge and best practice in this field are constantly changing. As new research and experience broaden our understanding, changes in research methods, professional practices, or medical treatment may become necessary.

Practitioners and researchers must always rely on their own experience and knowledge in evaluating and using any information, methods, compounds, or experiments described herein. In using such information or methods they should be mindful of their own safety and the safety of others, including parties for whom they have a professional responsibility.

With respect to any drug or pharmaceutical products identified, readers are advised to check the most current information provided (i) on procedures featured or (ii) by the manufacturer of each product to be administered, to verify the recommended dose or formula, the method and duration of administration, and contraindications. It is the responsibility of practitioners, relying on their own experience and knowledge of their patients, to make diagnoses, to determine dosages and the best treatment for each individual patient, and to take all appropriate safety precautions.

To the fullest extent of the law, neither the publisher nor the authors, contributors, or editors, assume any liability for any injury and/or damage to persons or property as a matter of products liability, negligence or otherwise, or from any use or operation of any methods, products, instructions, or ideas contained in the material herein.

ELSEVIER your source for books, journals and multimedia in the health sciences
www.elsevierhealth.com

Working together to grow libraries in developing countries
www.elsevier.com • www.bookaid.org

The publisher's policy is to use paper manufactured from sustainable forests

ISBN: 9780323353878
Printed in China
Last digit is the print number: 9 8 7 6 5 4 3

Content Strategist: *Charlotta Kryhl*
Content Development Specialist: *Helen Leng*
Project Manager: *Louisa Talbott*
Design: *Christian Bilbow*
Illustration Manager: *Amy Naylor*
Illustrator: *Jade Myers of Matrix Inc.*
Marketing Manager(s) (UK/USA): *Veronica Short*

Contents

Online contents

The accompanying Expert Consult website and eBook contain illustrative case videos detailing seizure semiology and simultaneous EEG data. Please visit www.expertconsult.com for access – details are available on the inside front cover of the printed text.

Foreword

Reading EEG is a skill that involves both science and art. Most of us learn by apprenticeship. If you are very lucky, you learn to read with an expert sitting in the chair next to you, helping you discover the logic and the beauty of the squiggles on the page. Slowly, these squiggles that initially seem incomprehensible begin to emerge as an unfolding story. Through interpretation of the EEG (if done correctly), much is revealed about the person being tested. With time, one learns to uncover hints and clues, like a detective, that lead to a correct interpretation.

I was fortunate enough to have had A. James Rowan sitting next to me as I learned to read EEG. Now with his primer, updated by Marcuse, Fields and Yoo, those learning to read for the first time can benefit from a simple, easy to follow, pragmatic guide that is perfect for carrying with you to have at your side as you learn to become comfortable with the EEG. Essential information is easy to find, and the pictures and diagrams beautifully illustrate the normal and abnormal EEG. The chapter on the technical aspects of the EEG is clear, simple and easy to follow. The illustrations of artifact have been carefully chosen, as have the normal variants and pathological epileptiform and non-epileptiform abnormalities. Each chapter provides just enough material to be helpful but not overwhelming, and there is a reference section for those seeking more in-depth information. The book will also be extremely useful to teachers of EEG, and I for one will be using the illustrations to train young encephalographers.

According to the dictionary, a primer is a book that "provides instruction in the rudiments or basic skills of a branch of knowledge". Those who master this primer will be well on their way to learning the art of EEG interpretation.

Jacqueline A French MD

Dedication

We dedicate this book to our patients (and yours as well): past, present, and future.

Preface to the second edition

"If I keep on saying to myself that I cannot do a certain thing, it is possible that I may end by really becoming incapable of doing it. On the contrary, if I have the belief that I can do it, I shall surely acquire the capacity to do it even if I may not have it at the beginning." – Mahatma Gandhi

With this book, we seek to lay the art of reading EEGs at your feet. We have built upon the structure of the first edition. We have added a chapter entitled *The normal EEG from neonates to adolescents*. All pictures of EEGs have been replaced, to give the readers up-to-date examples of normal and abnormal findings. In Chapter 5 we describe the typical EEG findings in all seizure types, electroclinical syndromes and other epilepsies as listed by the International League Against Epilepsy (ILAE).

Learning to understand an EEG is wonderful, and reporting those findings with standard nomenclature ensures that we all mean the same thing when we use the same word. This edition uses the 10-10 system of electrode placement and the nomenclature put forth by the American Clinical Neurophysiology Society (ACNS).

If you are a medical student with no intention of becoming a neurologist, we believe this primer will serve you well in understanding the EEG reports of both your outpatients and inpatients. If you are a neurologist or a neurology resident, we have included details which are useful to have at one's fingertips and easily forgotten (e.g., the meaning of subclinical rhythmic electroencephalographic discharges of adults).

As a companion to the print book, this edition has an online version, which includes a quiz for each chapter. Be warned, these questions are challenging. The answers are detailed and meant to help you integrate what you are learning of EEG with clinical care and clinical decision-making. Perhaps most importantly, we have created a video library of seizures. These can be watched with our annotations describing the seizure semiology and the electrographic findings, or you can choose to watch the seizures without the annotations to test your developing skill. We will be adding to the video library continually to build on your knowledge.

Learning the skill of electroencephalography may be challenging, it may be daunting, and it may not give us all the answers. However, it is a relatively inexpensive window into the workings of the brain, which often provides very valuable information for diagnosis, prognosis, and management of our patients.

We hope this primer will serve to increase your enthusiasm and dedication to the study of the brain, as this inquiry continues to nourish us as clinicians, teachers and researchers.

Lara V Marcuse MD (r)
Madeline C Fields MD (c)
Jiyeoun (Jenna) Yoo MD (l)

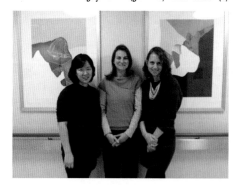

Origin and technical aspects of the EEG

ORIGIN OF THE EEG

The EEG records electrical activity from the cerebral cortex. Inasmuch as electrocortical activity is measured in microvolts (μV), it must be amplified by a factor of 1,000,000 in order to be displayed on a computer screen. Most of what we record is felt to originate from neurons, and there are a number of possible sources including action potentials, post-synaptic potentials (PSPs), and chronic neuronal depolarization. Action potentials induce a brief (10 ms or less) local current in the axon with a very limited potential field. This makes them unlikely candidates. PSPs are considerably longer (50–200 ms), have a much greater field, and thus are more likely to be the primary generators of the EEG. Long-term depolarization of neurons or even glia could also play a role and produce EEG changes.

In the normal brain an action potential travels down the axon to the nerve terminal, where a neurotransmitter is released. However, it is the synaptic potentials that are the most important source for the electroencephalogram. The resting membrane potential (electrochemical equilibrium) is typically −70 mV on the inside. At the post-synaptic membrane the neurotransmitter produces a change in membrane conductance and transmembrane potential. If the signal has an excitatory effect on the neuron it leads to a local reduction of the transmembrane potential (depolarization) and is called an excitatory post-synaptic potential (EPSP), typically located in the dendrites. Note that during an EPSP the inside of the neuronal membrane becomes more positive while the extracellular matrix becomes more negative. Inhibitory post-synaptic potentials (IPSPs) result in local hyperpolarization typically located on the cell body of the neuron. The combination of EPSPs and IPSPs induces currents that flow within and around the neuron with a potential field sufficient to be recorded on the scalp. The EEG is essentially measuring these voltage changes in the extracellular matrix. It turns out that the typical duration of a PSP, 100 ms, is similar to the duration of the average alpha wave. The posterior dominant rhythm (PDR), consisting of sinusoidal or rhythmic alpha waves, is the basic rhythmic frequency of the normal awake adult brain.

It is easy to understand how complex neuronal electrical activity generates irregular EEG signals that translate into seemingly random and ever-changing EEG waves. Less obvious is the physiological explanation of the rhythmic character of certain EEG patterns seen both in sleep and wakefulness. The mechanisms underlying EEG rhythmicity, although not completely understood, are mediated through two main processes. The first is the interaction between cortex and thalamus. The activity of thalamic pacemaker cells leads to rhythmic cortical activation. For example, the cells in the nucleus reticularis of the thalamus have the pacing properties responsible for the generation of sleep spindles. The second is based on the functional properties of large neuronal networks in the cortex that have an intrinsic capacity for rhythmicity. The result of both mechanisms is the creation of recognizable EEG patterns, varying in different areas of neocortex that allow us to make sense of the complex world of brain waves.

TECHNICAL CONSIDERATIONS

The essence of electroencephalography is the amplification of tiny currents into a graphic representation that can be interpreted. Of course, extracerebral potentials are likewise amplified (movements and the like), and these are many times the amplitude of electrocortical potentials. Thus, unless understood and corrected for, such interference or artifacts obscure the underlying EEG. Like the archeologist, the epileptologist seeks to fully understand artifacts in order to discern the truth. Later, we will discuss artifacts in detail and illustrate clearly their many guises. At this point we will consider the technical factors that are indispensable in obtaining an interpretable record.

ELECTRODES

Electrodes are simply the means by which the electrocortical potentials are conducted to the amplification apparatus. Essentially, standard EEG electrodes are small, non-reactive metal discs or cups applied to the scalp with a conductive paste. Several types of metals are used including gold, silver/silver chloride, tin, and platinum. Electrode contact must be firm in order to ensure low impedance (resistance to current flow), thus minimizing both electrode and environmental artifacts.

For long-term monitoring, especially if the patient is mobile, cup electrodes are affixed with collodion (a sort of glue), and a conductive gel is inserted between electrode and scalp through a small hole in the electrode itself. This procedure maintains recording integrity over prolonged periods.

Other types of electrodes are available including plastic, as well as needle electrodes. In fact, new plastic electrodes are MRI compatible. Needle electrodes, which in the past were often used in ICUs, have been redeveloped and consist of a painless (really!) subdermal electrode.

ELECTRODE PLACEMENT

Electrode placement is standardized in the United States and indeed in most other nations. This allows EEGs performed in one laboratory to be interpreted in another. The general problem is to record activity from various parts of the cerebral cortex in a logical, interpretable manner. Thanks to Dr. Herbert Jasper, a renowned electroencephalographer at the Montreal Neurological Institute, we have a logical, generally accepted system of electrode placement: the 10-20 International System of Electrode Placement (Figure 1-1). The numbering has been slightly modified since the last edition to a 10-10 system (Figure 1-2). The system was modified so that if additional electrodes are to be placed on the scalp, there is a logical numbering system with which to do so.

Both the 10-10 and the 10-20 system depend on accurate measurements of the skull, utilizing several distinctive landmarks. Essentially, a measurement of the skull is taken in three planes – sagittal, coronal, and horizontal. The summation of all the electrodes in any given plane will equal 100%. Electrodes designated with odd numbers are on the left; those with even numbers are on the right. Standard electrode designations and placement should be memorized during the student's first day of his or her elective (Table 1-1).

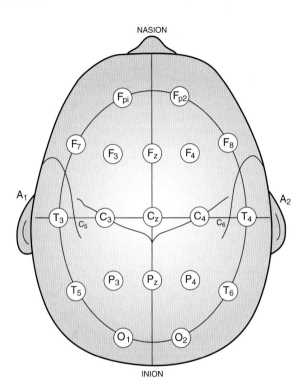

Figure 1-1 10-20 system. A single-plane projection of the head showing all standard positions and the locations of the Rolandic and Sylvian fissures. The outer circle was drawn at the level of the nasion and inion. The inner circle represents the temporal line of electrodes.

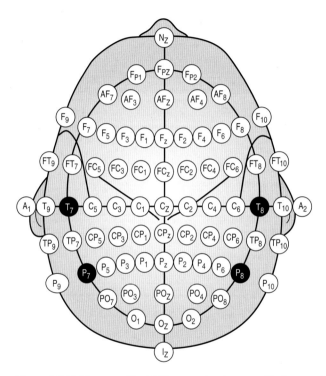

Figure 1-2 10-10 system. The 10-20 system has been modified to standardize a method for adding more electrodes.

Table 1-1 Standard electrode designations

Left	Right	Electrode
		Parasagittal/supra-sylvian electrodes
Fp1	Fp2	Frontopolar, located on the forehead – postscripted numbers are different than other electrodes in this sagittal line (3,4)
F3	F4	Mid-frontal
C3	C4	Central – roughly over the central sulcus
P3	P4	Parietal
O1	O2	Occipital-postscripted numbers are different from other electrodes in this sagittal line (3,4)
		Lateral/temporal electrodes
F7	F8	Inferior frontal/anterior temporal
T7	T8	Mid-temporal – formerly T3, T4
P7	P8	Posterior temporal/parietal – formerly T5,T6
		Other electrodes
Fz, Cz, Pz		Midline electrodes: Frontal, central and parietal.
A1	A2	Earlobe electrodes. Often used as reference electrodes from contralateral side. Of note, they record ipsilateral mid-temporal activity.
LLC	RUC	Left lower canthus/right upper canthus (placed on the lower and upper outer corners of the eyes). These electrodes are used to detect eye movements and can help distinguish eye movements from brain activity. Sometimes designated LOC, ROC.

How to measure for electrode placement

Sagittal plane: The sagittal measurement starts at the nasion (the depression at the top of the nose) over the top the head to the inion (the prominence in the midline at the base of the occiput). With a red wax pencil, mark the point above the nasion that is 10% of the total measurement (Fpz) and the point above the inion that also is 10% of the total (Oz). These locations are used as coordinates to help identify the other designated electrode destinations. Divide and mark the remaining 80% into four segments, each 20% of the total measurement. The first 20% point is Fz, the second Cz and the third Pz – the midline electrodes (z = zero). The final 20% is the distance between Pz and your point 10% above the inion (Oz). Thus, the total is 100% (Figure 1-3A).

Coronal plane: The coronal plane extends from the point anterior to the tragus (the cartilaginous protrusion at the front of the external ear) to the same point on the opposite side, making sure that the tape measure traverses the Cz point on the sagittal measurement. The intersection of the halfway (50%) points of the sagittal and coronal measurements is the location of the vertex and thus the Cz electrode. The first 10% points up from the tragus define T7 and T8, the mid-temporal electrodes. The next 20% points then define C3 and C4, the central

electrodes. The remaining 20% segments represent the distance from C3 to Cz and Cz to C4 (Figure 1-3B).

Horizontal plane: The trickiest measurements are in the horizontal plane. The horizontal plane is generated with a measurement from Fpz to T7 to Oz on the left and from Fpz to T8 to Oz on the right. Fp1 and Fp2 are placed on either side of Fpz, both a distance of 5% of the total horizontal circumference from Fpz. Similarly, O1 and O2 are placed at a 5% distance of the total horizontal circumference from Oz. The distances from Fp1 to F7 to T7 to P7 to O1 on the left and from Fp2 to F8 to T8 to P8 to O2 on the right are all 10% of the total horizontal circumference (Figure 1-3C).

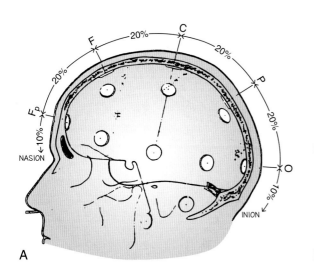

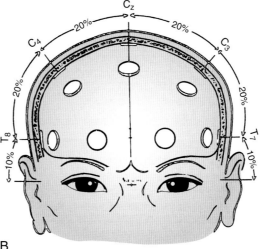

Figure 1-3 Measurements in the 10-10 system in the (**A**) sagittal, (**B**) coronal, and (**C**) horizontal plane. (**A**) Lateral view of the skull to show the method of measurement from the nasion to inion at the mid-line. Fp is the frontal pole position, F is the frontal line of electrodes, C is the central line, P is the parietal line, and O is the occipital line. Percentages indicate proportions of the total measurement from the nasion to the inion. The central line is 50% of this distance. (**B**) Frontal view of the skull showing the coronal measurements.

Finally, F3 and F4 are defined by the halfway points between F7 and Fz on the left and F8 and Fz on the right. Similarly, P3 and P4 are defined by the halfway points between P7 and Pz on the left and P8 and Pz on the right.

An observation: The F7 and F8 electrodes are probably placed too high for optimal definition of anterior temporal activity. Likewise, the P7 and P8 electrodes are probably too high for good definition of posterior temporal activity. Thus, it is possible to logically place additional electrodes (F9/F10, T9/T10, and P9/P10), which are placed 10% inferior to the standard (F7/8, T7/8, P7/8, respectively) electrodes. In some laboratories, these additional electrodes are routinely used.

In the 10-10 system, there are remaining electrode positions in the 10% intermediate lines between the existing standard coronal and sagittal lines. Best to look at Figure 1-2 while reading the next several sentences. Coronally, these electrode positions are named by combining the designation of the coronal lines anterior and posterior. For example, the coronal line between the parietal (P) and occipital (O) chain is designated PO. The only exception is in the first intermediate coronal line, which is named AF (anterior frontal) rather than FpF or FF. In the sagittal line, the same postscript numbers are used; for example, AF3, F3, FC3, C3, CP3, P3, and PO3. From the midline moving laterally the postscript begins at z followed by the numbers 1, 3, 5, 7, 9 on the left and 2, 4, 6, 8, 10 on the right. We now have the 10-10 system where each letter appears on only one coronal line and each postscripted number on a sagittal line (*except for* Fp1/Fp2 and O1/O2). The 10-10 system locates each electrode at the intersection of a specific coronal (identified by the letter) and sagittal (identified by the number) line.

While the 10-10 system may sound ever so slightly complicated, in practice it is quite easily carried out. Nonetheless, there is nothing like actually measuring and placing the electrodes yourself under the guidance of an experienced EEG technologist. We recommend that all

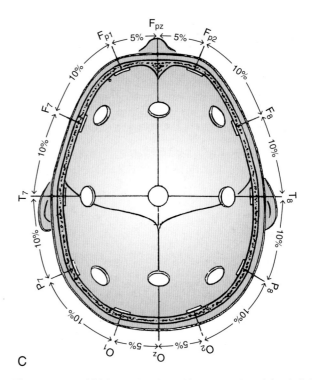

C

Figure 1-3, cont'd (C) Superior view with cross-section of the skull through the temporal line of electrodes.

residents perform at least two to three supervised EEGs during their EEG rotations. Fellows should do more until they are confident in their ability to measure accurately and apply electrodes properly.

POTENTIAL FIELDS

Before discussing how we display the electrical information recorded by the electrodes, the reader should understand the concept of the potential field. The summation of IPSPs and EPSPs in a neuronal net creates electrical currents that flow in and around the cells. The flow of current creates a field that spreads out from the origin of an electrical event (such as a spike or slow wave), much the same as the concentric rings created on a glassy pond when one tosses a pebble onto its surface. Potential fields are usually oval in shape and may be quite restricted or very widespread. The field's effect diminishes as the distance from the source increases. This means that events producing maximal voltage on a particular electrode will affect adjacent electrodes as well, but to a lesser extent as the potential wanes from the point of origin (Figure 1-4).

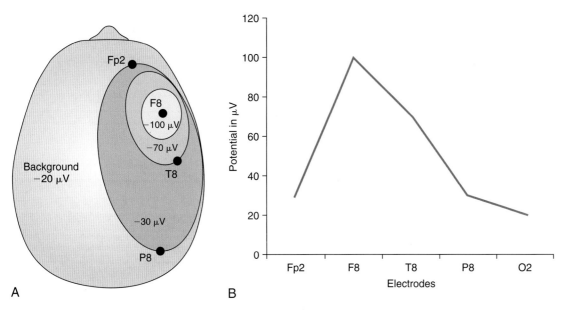

A   B

Figure 1-4 A potential field. (**A**) The figure illustrates a maximum negative potential of -100 μV at F8. The field spreads to involve T8 at a lower potential of −70 μV and then to Fp2 and P8 at −30 μV. The background averages −20 μV. (**B**) Another way to depict the same data. Note the steep rise from Fp2 to F8, declining successively to T8 and P8.

AMPLIFICATION

Easiest to understand is the simple amplifier. Input from a single active electrode is conducted to the amplifier and compared with ground (earth). Thus, the output consists of the potential difference between the active electrode and ground. Electrocortical potentials, as well as other environmental potentials affecting the electrode (e.g., 60 Hz interference), are displayed in the output. In differential amplification, signals from two active leads are conducted to the amplifier, thus measuring the potential difference between the two (Figure 1-5). In this case, any signal that affects both inputs identically (say 60 Hz) will result in no potential difference and thus will not be displayed or be much reduced. This phenomenon is termed in-phase cancellation.

We are now in a position to consider methods of recording electrocortical potentials so that we can make sense of them. Recalling that amplifiers record potential difference between two incoming signals, we can record the potential difference between two electrodes on the scalp (bipolar recording). On the other hand, we can record the potential difference between a scalp electrode and another point (the reference) that, ideally, is unaffected by cerebral potentials or other interference (referential recording). Unfortunately, it is virtually impossible to achieve this ideal, but certain references (e.g., the ears) are quite serviceable. These two types of recording, along with their advantages and disadvantages, are discussed below.

BIPOLAR RECORDING

Bipolar recordings electronically link successive electrodes (known as a chain or line). The voltage at one electrode is compared with the voltage affecting adjacent electrodes (potential difference). Each amplifier has two inputs, I and II. By convention, the rules for understanding the display are:

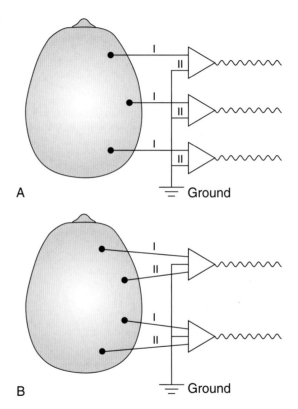

Figure 1-5 (A) Simple amplifier. Input from each active electrode is compared with ground. **(B)** Differential amplifier. Here, potential difference is measured between two active electrodes.

If input I becomes negative with respect to input II, there is an upward deflection.

If input II becomes negative with respect to input I, there is a downward deflection.

Contrary to our well-used Cartesian coordinate system, the convention in neurophysiology is that an upward deflection is negative and a downward deflection is positive.

In the simplest example, consider a spike with a very limited potential field involving only T8 (Figure 1-6). The electrode pairs (or derivations) in this case are F8–T8 and T8–P8. F8–T8 is Channel 1, and T8–P8 is Channel 2. In Channel 1 T8 is in input II, and in Channel 2 T8 is in input I. The voltage at T8 (–100 μV) is compared with the background activity at F8 and P8 (–20 μV). Therefore, in this example:

Channel 1: F8–T8 = –20 μV– (–100 μV) = 80 μV (downward deflection)

Channel 2: T8–P8 = (–100 μV) – (–20 μV) = –80 μV (upward deflection)

In this case, the adjacent channels containing the T8 electrode record the same potential but in opposite directions. This creates the phase reversal. Most spike discharges at the surface are negative in sign, and negative phase reversals resemble two sharp points touching or nearly touching. Channels 1 and 2 are displaying the same potential but with opposite deflections. Again, this is phase reversal – the localization principle of bipolar recording.

Let us now analyze the display when a spike at F8 has a wider potential field that also affects Fp2 and T8 (Figure 1-7A). In Channel 1, the voltage at Fp2 (–50 μV) is compared with the voltage at F8 (–100 μV). In Channel 2, the voltage at F8 (–100 μV) is compared with the voltage at T8 (–50 μV). In Channel 3, the voltage at T8 (–50 μV) is compared

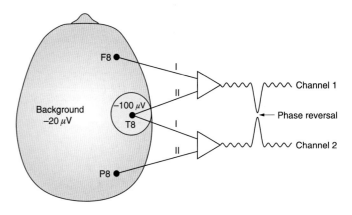

Figure 1-6 Principle of bipolar localization. The figure depicts a spike discharge of –100 μV at T8. The potential is conducted to input II in the first amplifier and to input I in the second amplifier. Other electrodes are not affected by the event. The result is known as a phase reversal.

to the voltage P8, which is unaffected by the spike at F8 but is recording the background activity (–20 μV). In Channel 4, the voltage at P8 is compared with O2, both unaffected by the F8 spike. Thus, there is no potential difference and no deflection.

Channel 1: Fp2–F8 = (–50 μV) – (–100 μV) = 50 μV (downward deflection)

Channel 2: F8–T8 = (–100 μV) – (–50 μV) = –50 μV (upward deflection)

Channel 3: T8–P8 = (–50 μV) – (–20 μV) = –30 μV (a smaller upward deflection)

Channel 4: P8–O2 = (–20 μV) – (–20 μV) = 0 μV (no deflection)

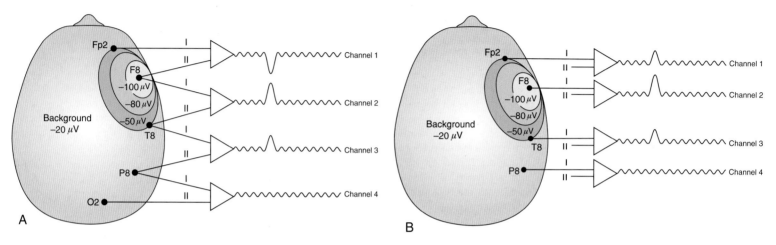

Figure 1-7 (A) Phase reversal in longitudinal bipolar montage. Here, a spike of −100 μV at F8 spreads to involve Fp2 and T8, each at −50 μV. The potential difference between F8 and the other two electrodes is 50 μV. The display demonstrates a phase reversal at F8 (Channels 1 and 2) with representation of the spike in Channel 3 (the potential difference between T8 and P8 is −30 μV). **(B)** Referential montage. The same spike displayed in a referential montage. In a referential montage, each electrode is compared to a reference electrode. The potential at the active electrode is conducted to input I of each amplifier. The reference electrode is conducted to input II. The amplitude of the displayed spike is proportional to the voltage at each active electrode.

Other channels (e.g., F4–C4 and C4–P4) may be affected by the declining potential field generated at F8. Thus, phase reversals at lower amplitude would be recorded at these sites. Note that these considerations apply to any potential at any point on the scalp.

REFERENTIAL RECORDING

In referential recording the amplifiers are not linked as in bipolar recording. Signals from each of the scalp electrodes are conducted to input I of the associated amplifier, while signals from the reference are conducted to input II. Thus, in referential recording, we record the potential difference between a particular scalp electrode and a referential electrode. Reference montages produce a higher amplitude EEG recording because of the longer interelectrode distances. Theoretically, the reference can be located anywhere, but there are practical considerations. A reference placed at any distant point will be contaminated with ambient electrical noise, 60 Hz artifact (50 Hz in Europe). A reference placed on, say, the shoulder or chest would also pick up high-voltage EKG artifact. Interference from an EKG would render the EEG unreadable. The ears are relatively free from both these artifacts, although it must be said that EKG is sometimes a contaminant at the ear electrodes. Moreover, due to the proximity of the ears to the mid-temporal lobes, the ears do pick up cerebral activity.

Now, utilizing the ears as a contralateral reference, let us compare the voltage of an event occurring at F8 with that at a contralateral ear reference, A1 (Figure 1-7B). In this example we will assume that A1 is recording the same as the background at –20 μV. Here we have a spike discharge with an amplitude of –100 μV at F8. The potential field of the spike spreads to Fp2 and T8 with an amplitude of –50 μV. Beyond these points there is no representation of the field associated with the spike.

Channel 1: Fp2–A1 = (–50 μV) – (–20 μV) = –30 μV (small upward deflection)

Channel 2: F8–A1 = (–100 μV) – (–20 μV)= –80 μV (big upward deflection)

Channel 3: T8–A1 = (–50 μV) – (–20 μV) = –30 μV (small upward deflection)

Channel 4: P8–A1 = (–20 μV) – (–20 μV) = 0 μV (no deflection)

In referential recording, the localization principle is amplitude. That is, the electrode recording the greatest amplitude of the wave in question, in this case a spike at F8, defines the focus.

References other than the ears are also in common use. One is the vertex (Cz), often used in a referential montage to complement the ear reference. The astute reader will recognize that the vertex resides in a sea of cerebral activity. Thus, the background of the EEG recorded by the vertex electrode will be input II of all channels. As long as this is recognized, one is able to determine the location of a waveform that stands out from the background (e.g., a spike or delta wave).

A note on ear and vertex referential recording: A recorded event (spike, slow wave) is best represented when the reference is distant from the exploring electrode. Considering the ipsilateral ear reference (A1 or A2), the ear is close to the midtemporal electrodes T7 or T8. When examining a spike at T7, the ipsilateral ear reference (A1) is not an appropriate choice, as the potentials at T7 and A1 are very similar. A vertex reference or a contralateral ear reference (A2) is more appropriate for the examination of that T7 spike. Similarly, a spike that is maximal at C3 will be ill served by placing it in a reference montage using the Cz electrode, as the reference and the active electrode are too close together. For a C3 spike, either ear electrode would be an appropriate reference. The reference chosen for a particular spike should be as distant as possible from that spike.

A widely used reference is the common average reference. In this scheme, the voltage of an event occurring under a particular electrode (input I) is compared with the average voltage recorded by all the electrodes on the scalp (input II). This creates a situation in which a focal spike discharge, maximal at T8, will result in an upward deflection at T8 as T8 will be more electronegative than the average reference. Neighboring electrodes involved in the field, for example at F8, will have upward deflections as well, but these will be lower in amplitude. Note that the upward deflections thus recorded define the potential field of the event. Electrodes not involved in the negative spike discharge at T8 will be relatively electropositive compared with the average reference and thus will have a downward deflection (Figure 1-8).

We now present the paradox of bipolar recording and stress how important it is to use the various montages in a complementarily fashion. The paradox is a result of the previously mentioned in-phase cancellation – that is, potentials that are equal in the two inputs of an amplifier are isoelectric in the display. In other words, there is no potential

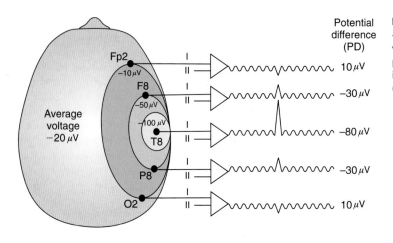

Potential
difference
(PD)

10 μV

−30 μV

−80 μV

−30 μV

10 μV

Figure 1-8 The common average reference. Recording of a spike discharge at T8 of −100 μV. The reference (going into input II at each channel) is the common average voltage, which in this case is −20 μV. In Channels 2, 3, and 4 the amplitude is proportional to the recorded voltage at each electrode. The downward deflection in channels 1 and 5 is due to the fact that Fp2 and O2 are relatively electropositive (−10 μV) compared with the average voltage (−20 μV).

difference! The unwary, when examining Channels 2 and 3 of Figure 1-9A, might conclude that little if anything is occurring at F8, T8, and P8. On the other hand, when one looks at the same situation with a referential recording, it becomes clear that the maximum abnormality underlies those very electrodes (Figure 1-9B).

MONTAGE SELECTION

Montage refers to the pattern of systematic linkage of the scalp electrodes designed to obtain a logical display of the electrical activity. Unlike the 10-10 system of electrode placement described earlier, there is no international standard of montages to be used in EEG laboratories. Certain montages, however, are in widespread use. In bipolar recording the longitudinal arrangement is perhaps the most popular (known in the trade as the "double banana," and by some as the Queen Square

montage) (Figure 1-10A). **Note:** arrows are often used in North America for convenience: the tail of the arrow indicates input I; the point of the arrow input II.

Adjacent electrodes are connected from front to back, including the temporal (lateral) chain and the parasagittal (supra-sylvian) chain. The EEG is displayed in various ways. In this example, the four channels of the temporal chain on one side are followed by the temporal channels on the opposite side. Similarly, the four channels of the parasagittal chain also alternate. In North America, the left side is written out first followed by the right. In Europe the opposite is the case. Some laboratories write out the eight channels of left-sided electrodes followed by the right-sided electrodes. Still others prefer alternating homologous channels, for example, Fp1 → F7; Fp2 → F8, and so on. Overall, the latter tends to be a bit more confusing – but electroencephalographers experienced with a particular electrode arrangement have no difficulty.

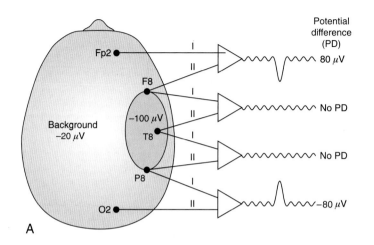
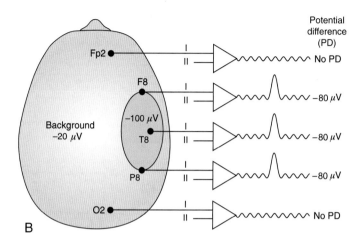

Figure 1-9 The paradox of bipolar recording. (**A**) Representation of a –100 µV spike that affects F8, T8, and P8 equally. Inasmuch as there is no potential difference between F8–T8 and T8–P8, the spike is not recorded in Channels 2 and 3 and gives the impression that there is no abnormality at T8. (**B**) Same discharge in referential recording. Note equal deflection in Channels 2, 3, and 4. The true picture is thus displayed.

A second popular arrangement is the transverse bipolar montage. This links adjacent electrodes in transverse chains, starting anteriorly and progressing posteriorly. Each chain starts with the left side and progresses to the right (i.e., F7 → F3 → Fz → F4 → F8). The transverse montage is particularly well suited to record abnormalities occurring at or near the vertex (e.g., midline spikes) (Figure 1-10B). One additional bipolar montage comes to mind: the circumferential montage. As the name implies, the circumferential montage encircles the head and is particularly useful for examining spikes and sharp waves, which occur at the end of the longitudinal bipolar chain: Fp1, Fp2, O1 or O2 (Figures 1-10C and 1-11).

With respect to referential recording, the recording is usually displayed in both A-P and transverse arrangements, reprising commonly used bipolar montages. A variety of other montages are employed at the discretion of the individual electroencephalographer. The idea, in short, is to highlight certain areas of interest in the best possible way. If the student is familiar with the 10-10 system and is apprised of the montage, he or she should have no difficulty in interpreting the record.

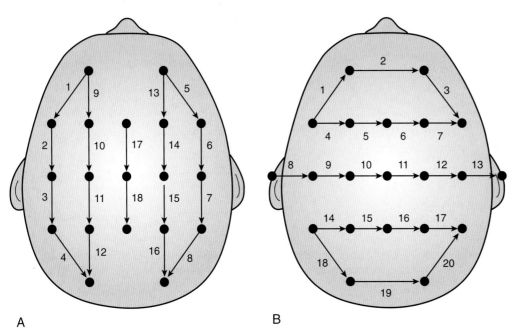

A

B

Figure 1-10 (A) A typical longitudinal bipolar montage. The numbers refer to channels, reflecting voltage difference between two electrodes. Both temporal and supra-sylvian chains alternate from left to right. The arrows represent the inputs to each amplifier. The tail is in input I and the arrow is in input II. **(B)** A transverse bipolar montage. The chains run from left to right, beginning anteriorly and proceeding posteriorly. Note that the midline electrodes are incorporated into the second, third, and fourth chains, thus allowing good representation of midline events.

In the era of digital EEG, specific montage selection by the technologist is not as critical as it was in the analog days. All recording is actually done referentially. The software allows display of recorded potentials in any desired montage. Thus, the technician and reader can now easily switch from one montage to another to examine the characteristics of a particular phenomenon. A low-amplitude temporal spike during bipolar recording can rapidly be inspected on a referential montage with the flick of the computer mouse.

In summary, the technologist may record an EEG in a set sequence of montages but the reviewing electroencephalographer can review the EEG in any montage desired. Furthermore, a given page or discharge can be examined in a variety of montages to help understand its meaning. Much as we would circle a complex sculpture in a museum, we circle an EEG wave by using different montages. Remember, the central idea is to maximize the opportunity to display an abnormality for optimal recognition.

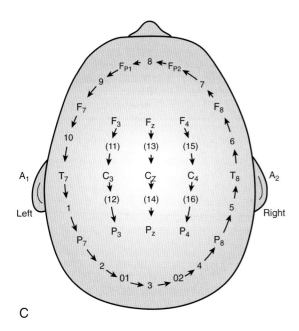

C

Figure 1-10, cont'd (**C**) Circumferential bipolar montage.

OVERVIEW OF ELECTRONICS

We often say that the EEG display can be manipulated at will and made to demonstrate a severe abnormality or to show a normal pattern. This manipulation refers to changing the electronic circuitry with the press of a button in order to alter sensitivity, filtration, and timebase.

Clearly, some order was required so that EEGs obtained in one laboratory are easily interpretable at another. For many years nearly all laboratories in North America, and indeed in many laboratories throughout the world, have used similar electronic settings for routine work. Following is a brief discussion of the most important recording parameters.

Calibration

Calibration is a way to accurately measure EEG potentials by administrating a standard signal through each amplifier. Once this is performed, the voltage of an EEG potential is compared against this known voltage. Calibration is currently built into the software of most digital EEG systems and is performed automatically. Additionally, an impedance check should appear at the start of every recording. The impedance check is a way of establishing the integrity of each electrode. Impedances should not exceed 5 kohms.

Display

In most North American and many European laboratories the standard display timebase is 30 mm/sec with 10 seconds of EEG per display. There is nothing magic about the number – in fact, some laboratories (particularly in Europe) prefer a timebase of 15 mm/sec. The appearance of the EEG is considerably altered in the latter case (i.e., the alpha rhythm at 30 mm/sec looks like rhythmic beta activity at 15 mm/sec). The important point is that the reader knows what timebase is selected. It should be said that there are instances when use of a shorter timebase is quite useful (e.g., in the identification of periodicity, or even rhythmicity of a particular phenomenon [e.g., in ICUs or for neonatal EEGs]). Likewise, increasing the timebase to, say, 60 mm/sec may allow one to analyze more accurately wave configuration, particularly when a phenomenon is "crowded" as in grouped spikes.

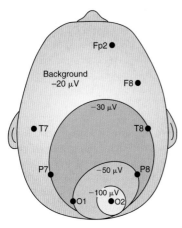

Figure 1-11 Occipital spike. Spike discharges at the "end of chain (Fp1, Fp2, O1, O2)" can be easy to miss in the standard longitudinal bipolar montage. Here, a right occipital (O2) spike discharge is displayed at –100 μV. (**A**) In a standard longitudinal bipolar montage, the deflection is always downward. (**B**) The discharge can be confirmed by placing it in a circumferential bipolar montage. Phase reversal at O2 confirms the spike maximum at this location.

Longitudinal bipolar montage	Potential difference (PD)	Circumferential posterior halo	Potential difference (PD)
Fp2-F8	No PD	T8-P8	20 μV
F8-T8	10 μV	P8-O2	50 μV
T8-P8	20 μV	O2-O1	–50 μV
P8-O2	50 μV	O1-P7	–20 μV

A   B

Sensitivity

The sensitivity of each channel refers to the amplitude of the display produced by the received signal. The measurement is expressed in voltage per deflection. Standard sensitivity is 7 μV/mm.

Sensitivity may be altered for any particular channel depending on the specific need. For example, the sensitivity of a channel recording the EKG would have to be decreased due to the much higher voltage of this signal (measured in millivolts). In general, the sensitivity of all channels recording the EEG may be changed simultaneously by a stepped gain control. For example, one might wish to increase sensitivity in situations where the general voltage of the EEG is low. Similarly, some EEG phenomena reach very high voltages (e.g., generalized spike-wave discharges), requiring a decrease in sensitivity (15 μV/mm) in order to properly analyze the waveforms. Please note, raising the gain from, for example, 7 μV to 15 μV is the same thing as lowering the sensitivity, and the EEG will appear lower in amplitude.

High-frequency filters (HFFs) or low pass filters

This circuit attenuates undesirable high frequencies (e.g., muscle action potentials) and passes low frequencies (Figure 1-12A). In an HFF circuit, the input signal is placed across the combination of a resistor and a

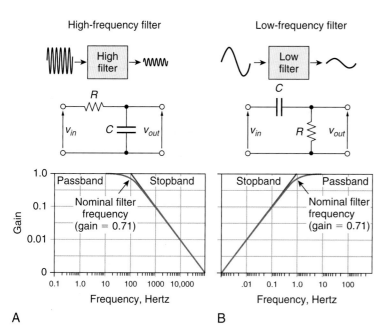

Figure 1-12 (A) High-frequency filter. In a high-frequency filter, the output voltage for high frequencies is lower than the input voltage for high frequencies. In the log–log graph, frequencies below the cutoff are unchanged while frequencies above the cutoff are attenuated. (**B**) Low-frequency filter. In a low-frequency filter, the output voltage for low frequencies is lower than the input voltage for low frequencies. In the log–log graph frequencies above the cutoffs are unchanged while frequencies below the cutoff are attenuated. (Adapted with permission from Lippincott Williams & Wilkins/Wolters Kluwer Health: Schomer, Lopes da Silva, Niedermeyer's Electroencephalography, 2010.)

capacitor in series and the output signal is measured across the capacitor alone (Figure 1-12A). At high frequencies, the impedance of any capacitor is low. Measuring output across the capacitor with a high frequency will be essentially zero, as the voltage does not change, so the potential difference is zero. The standard HF setting is 70 Hz. Other standard settings are 35 Hz and 15 Hz, the latter severely attenuating a broad range of high frequencies. As a practical matter, recording at a HFF setting of 15 Hz should not be employed save in rare and unusual circumstances. An unwanted consequence would be a marked attenuation of spike potentials. Unfortunately, the authors have inspected EEGs from outside sources in which an HFF setting of 15 Hz was used throughout. Such records look "clean" but fail to convey needed information. Don't do it.

Low-frequency filters (LFFs) or high-pass filters

In an LFF, there is marked attenuation of slow potentials below the cutoff frequency (such as those caused by sweat artifact, respirations, and tongue movement), with little effect on rapid potentials such as spikes or muscle artifacts. In an LFF circuit, the input signal is placed across the combination of a capacitor and a resistor in series and the output signal is measured across the resistor alone (Figure 1-12B). The impedance of any capacitor is very high at low frequencies. In this circuit arrangement, low-frequency input signals are essentially blocked. At higher frequencies, the impedance at the capacitor is low and the signal is measured across the resistor essentially unchanged from the input. The LFF is typically set at 1 Hz.

Notch filter

In addition, a notch filter setting of 60 Hz (US) or 50 Hz (Europe) is usually employed, selectively reducing environmental interference.

NOTES ON RECORDING THE EEG

Many special problems confront the technologist in his or her efforts to obtain an EEG that can be interpreted successfully by the electroencephalographer. We emphasize that the electroencephalographer is totally dependent on the quality of the recording – that is, regardless of the expertise of the reader, he or she is unable to use that expertise in the face of a technically inadequate tracing. The ability to properly place electrodes in conformity with the 10-10 International System (including, importantly, accurate measurements of electrode location) is critical if one is to compare electrical activity between the two hemispheres with accuracy. If epilepsy is suspected, the technologist should attempt to record drowsiness and sleep if possible. Moreover, because focal epileptiform activity is often activated by the interface between wake and drowsiness, the technologist should gently alert the drowsy patient on several occasions in an attempt to provoke spikes. Similarly, if a patient is sleeping at the onset of the test, he or she should be aroused after some minutes of recording. This ensures that a relative waking record is obtained. Unfortunately, sleep may obscure background abnormalities that are only evident when the patient is awake – a circumstance sometimes encountered in patients with dementia.

ARTIFACTS

Recognition of artifacts is one of the vexing and strangely satisfying aspects of EEG interpretation, as well as one of the most important. As a beginner, you may find the differentiation of artifacts from physiological phenomena quite difficult. A distinguishing characteristic of the experienced electroencephalographer is the ability reliably to recognize artifacts. For the most part the reader will soon master artifact recognition, particularly after understanding their characteristics and referring to the mini-atlas, and should not be too daunted by the seeming impossibility of this task!

Artifacts come in many different forms and have diverse causes. The major underlying problem is the enormous amplification required to record brain waves. As a result, amplified non-cerebral potentials – for example vigorous movements by the patient producing random excursions of the electrode leads – may render the EEG uninterpretable. Specific artifacts are detailed in Figures 1-13–1-30.

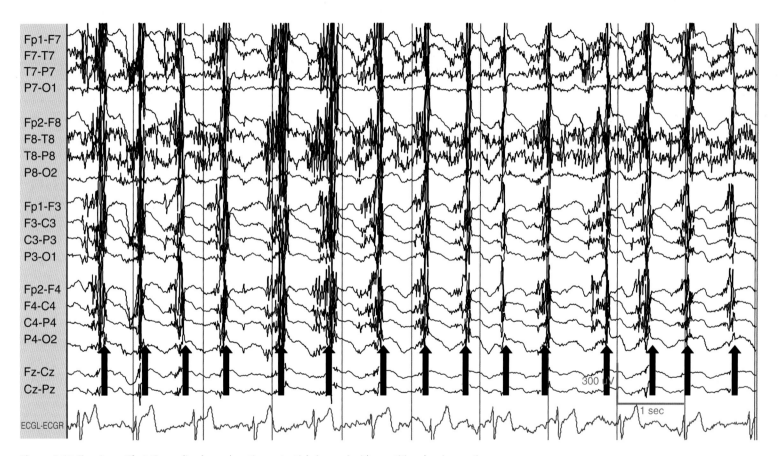

Figure 1-13 Chewing artifact. Generalized muscle action potentials (arrows) with repetitive chewing motions.

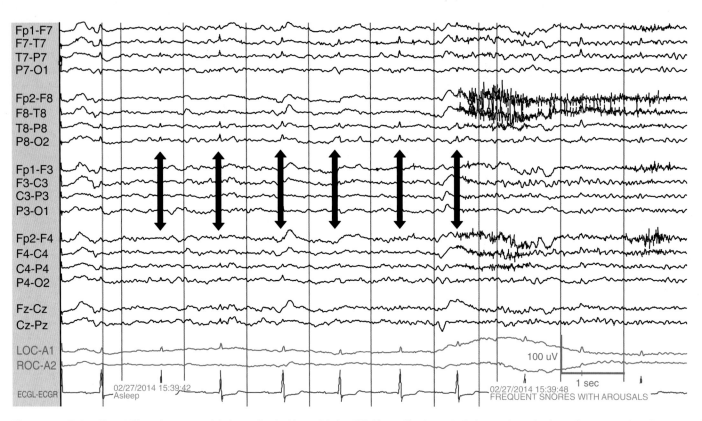

Figure 1-14 EKG artifact. Diffuse sharp potentials (arrows) coincident with the EKG. The artifact is particularly prominent in channels connected to the ears. It also may be diffuse. If there is no EKG monitor, and if the patient has atrial fibrillation or frequent premature contractions, the artifact may be confounding, be inconsistent, and masquerade as spike discharges. Look for phase relationships that do not comport with those of true spikes. EKG artifact is particularly prominent in the obese and those with hypertension.

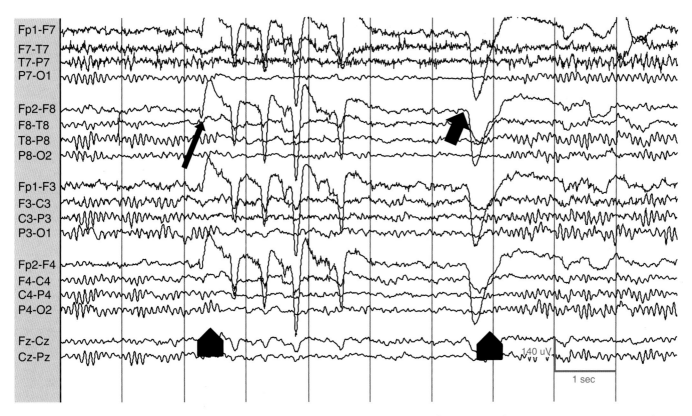

Figure 1-15 Eye blink artifact. High-voltage potentials, maximal in the frontal derivations. The deflection results from the cornea-retinal potential (the cornea is electropositive with respect to the retina, measured in millivolts), along with a minor contribution of the electroretinogram (ERG). During an eyeblink the globes turn slightly upward (Bell's phenomenon). Thus, the frontopolar electrodes become momentarily positive (to understand deflections, recall the rule for bipolar recording.) Figure shows eye opening (thin arrow), eye closure (thick arrow) and disappearance and reappearance of PDR (arrowheads).

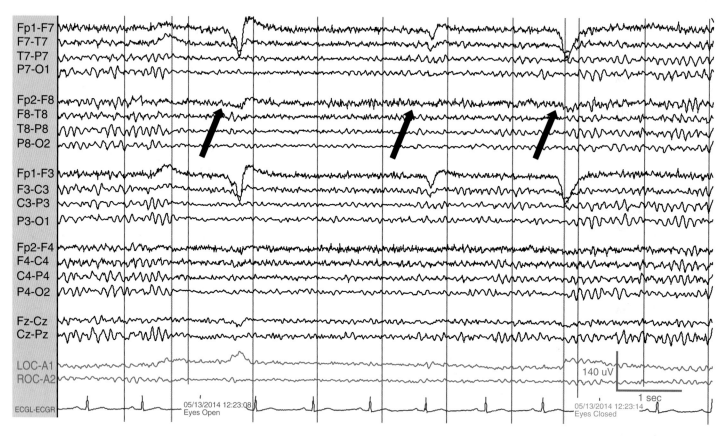

Figure 1-16 Prosthetic eye. In a patient with a right prosthetic eye, the blink artifact is expressed on only one side. Arrows point to missing right-sided eye blink artifact. One will also see limited eye blink potentials in those with a third nerve palsy.

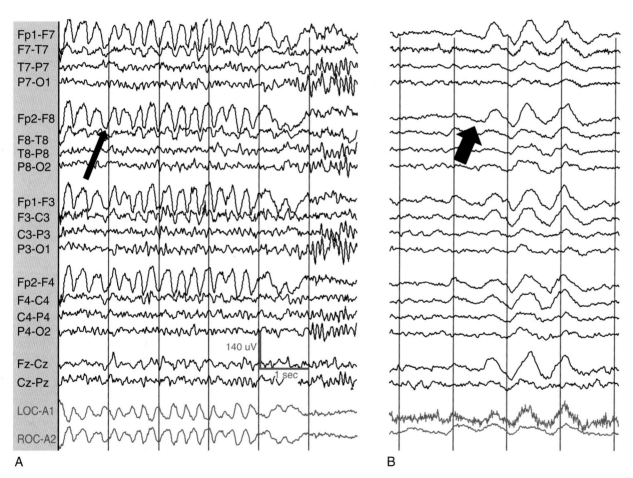

A

B

Figure 1-17 Eyelid flutter. In (**A**) eyelid-flutter produces a rhythmic bifrontal frequency, here at 3–4 Hz (thin arrow). Eye leads are out of phase as LOC is positioned on the left lower canthus and ROC is positioned on the right upper canthus. (**B**) Shows frontally predominant generalized rhythmic delta activity (GRDA) (thick arrow). Eye leads show synchronous (in phase) delta as both eye electrodes are anterior to the frontal lobe and recording very similar activity.

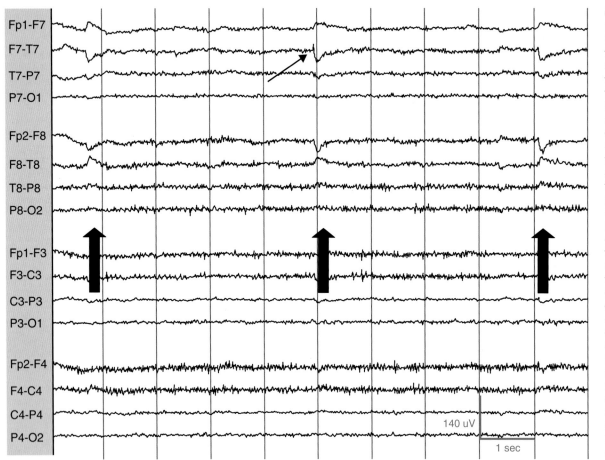

Fp1-F7	
F7-T7	
T7-P7	
P7-O1	
Fp2-F8	
F8-T8	
T8-P8	
P8-O2	
Fp1-F3	
F3-C3	
C3-P3	
P3-O1	
Fp2-F4	
F4-C4	
C4-P4	
P4-O2	

140 uV

1 sec

Figure 1-18 Lateral eye movement artifact (reading). Recognizable in the frontotemporal derivations as sharply contoured potentials that are out of phase. This figure shows three left saccades (thick arrows). When the eyes saccade to the left, the globe on the left approaches the left anterior temporal electrode (F7) while the right globe turns away from the right anterior temporal electrode (F8). A positive potential is therefore recorded at F7 and a negative potential at F8. (Remember, the cornea is positive with respect to the retina.) Thus, in bipolar recording, the resultant waveforms deviate away from each other in the two channels connected to F7, while the opposite is the case with the channels connected to F8. Note also that very rapid spike potentials may occur during lateral eye movements with potential maxima at the F7/F8 electrodes. These result from movements of the lateral rectus muscles and are known as lateral rectus spikes (thin arrow).

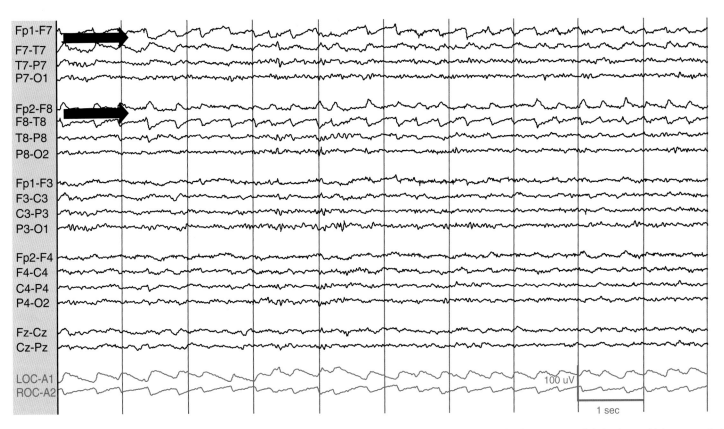

Figure 1-19 Nystagmus. In this patient with nystagmus, again there are sharply contoured potentials (arrows) in the frontotemporal derivations, which are out of phase. There is a rapid rise on the right side followed by a gradual fall, which is the corrective movement. The steeper positive phase reversal, seen here on the right, indicates the direction of the fast component of the nystagmus.

25

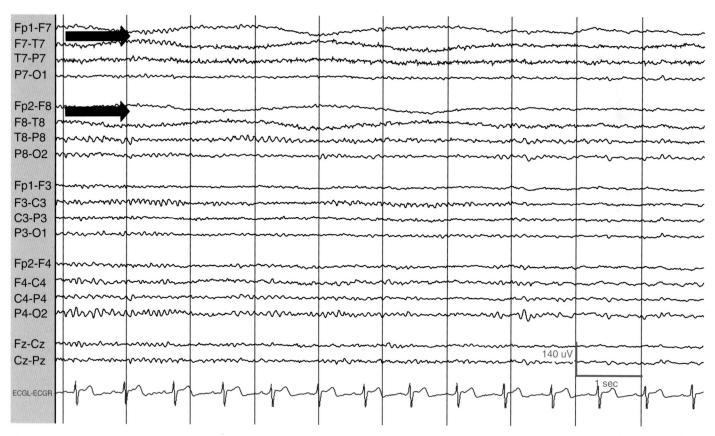

Figure 1-20 Roving eye movements. Slow, lateral eye movements during drowsiness that produce slow waves with alternating phase relationships in the frontotemporal derivations.

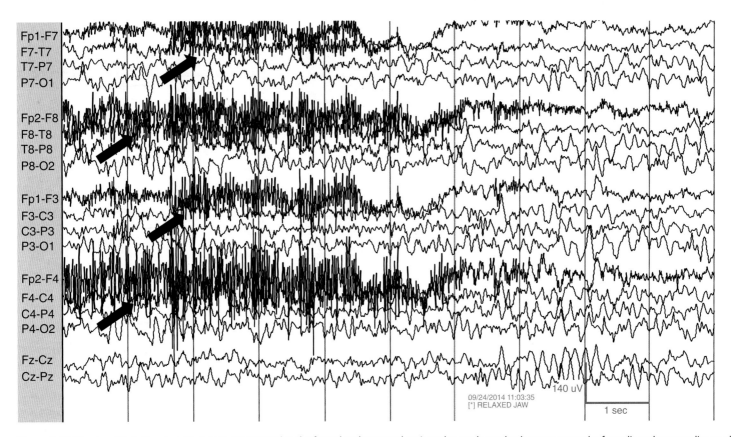

Figure 1-21 Muscle artifact. Muscle artifact (arrows) maximal in the frontal and temporal regions due to electrode placement over the frontalis and temporalis muscles. When the technician asks the patient to relax his jaw, the artifact dissipates. Muscle potentials are less than 20 ms, whereas cerebral spike potentials are longer, lasting 20–70 ms.

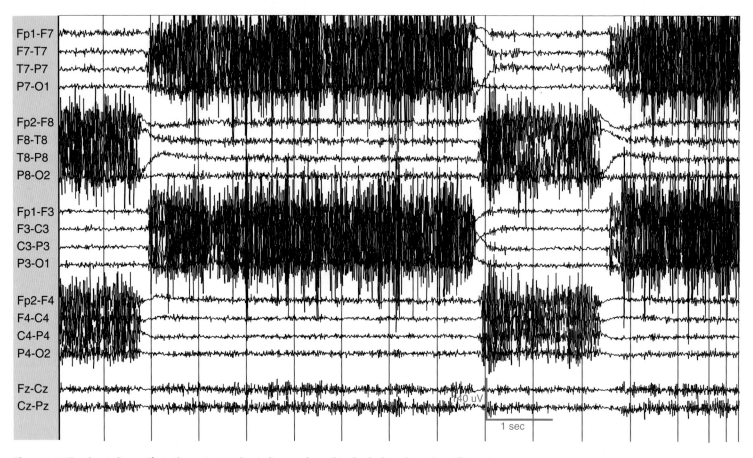

Figure 1-22 Tooth grinding artifact. Alternating tooth grinding produces this checkerboard muscle artifact pattern.

28

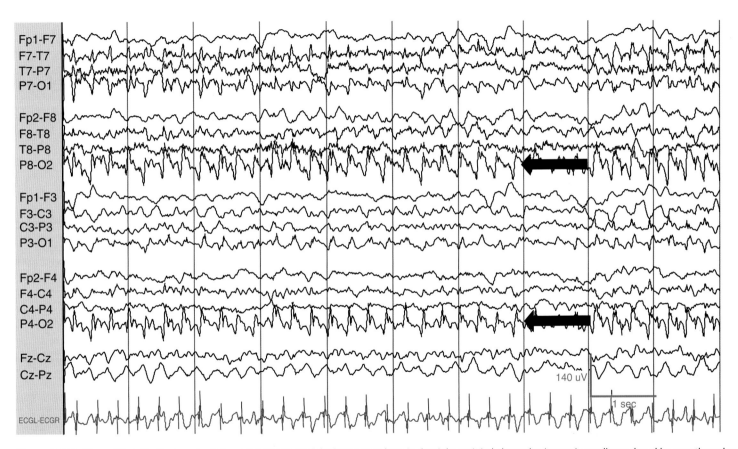

Figure 1-23 Patting artifact. Rhythmic potentials resembling an ictal discharge seen here in the right occipital electrodes (arrows), usually produced by a mother who holds her baby on her lap during the EEG. Notice the lack of a field anterior to the artifact.

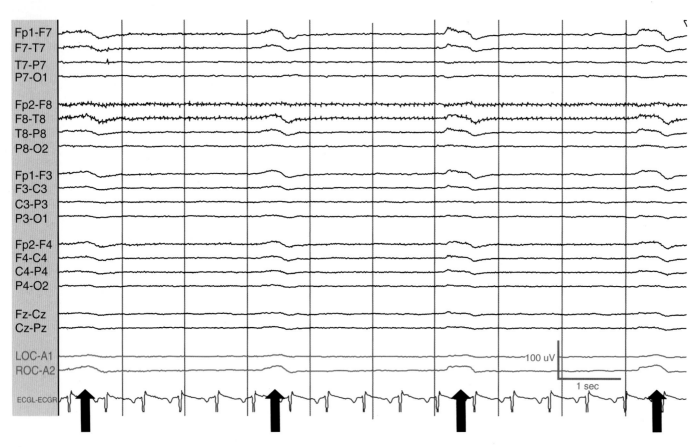

Figure 1-24 Ventilator artifact. Wide excursions (arrows) that may resemble delta waves. A check on the rhythmicity (usually in the range of 12 per min), along with a stereotyped waveform, makes the diagnosis. Note that the artifact, in cases where the patient overrides the respirator, may demonstrate irregularity. Amplitude can vary.

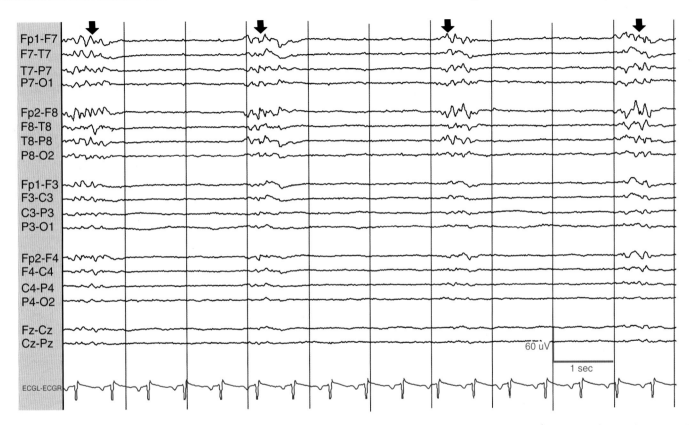

Figure 1-25 Respiratory artifact. Note the periodic bursts of sharply contoured theta/alpha frequency activity prominently seen over the anterior regions. In this patient (same patient as in Figure 1-23), this activity correlated with ventilator rate (chest rising movement) and disappeared with suction. This artifact is caused by the movement of fluids within the upper respiratory tract and/or the tube and can also occur irregularly in a patient overriding the respirator. Concomitant use of video and/or audio (sometimes you can hear gurgling sounds) can help to prevent misinterpreting these artifacts as cerebral rhythm.

31

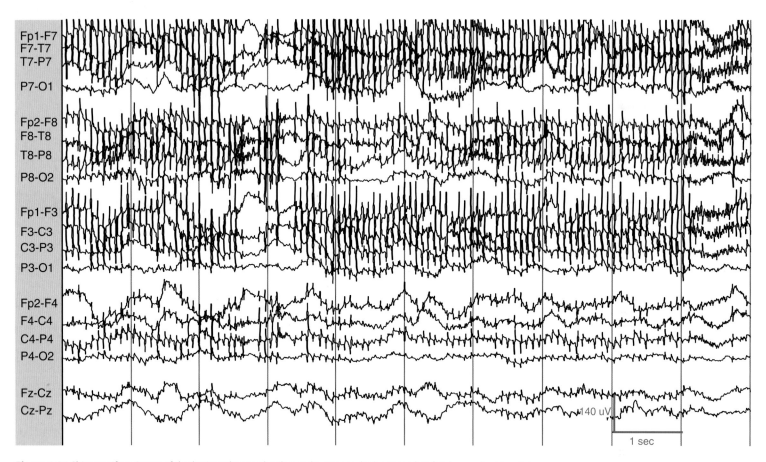

Figure 1-26 Shiver artifact. Bursts of rhythmic widespread spikes at 10–14 Hz, which are too brief to be cerebral in origin.

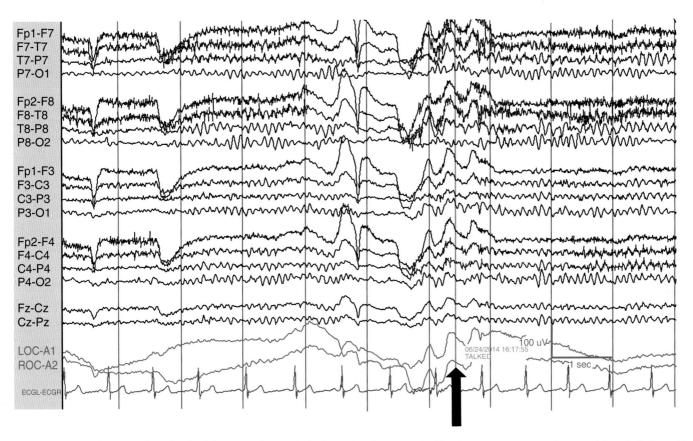

Figure 1-27 Glossokinetic artifact. The tip of the tongue is negatively charged, and movement of the tongue can cause synchronous delta activity (arrow) in the frontal derivations.

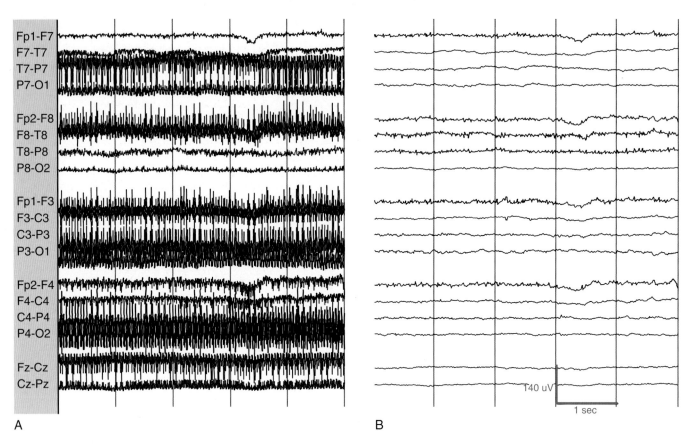

A

B

Figure 1-28 60 Hz artifact. Rhythmic frequency at 60 Hz (or 50 Hz in Europe) secondary to nearby electrical apparatus or poor grounding, usually expressed because of high electrode impedance but sometimes (particularly in the ICU) difficult to eliminate. (**A**) Shows EEG with a great deal of 60 Hz artifact. In (**B**) the notch filter has been applied.

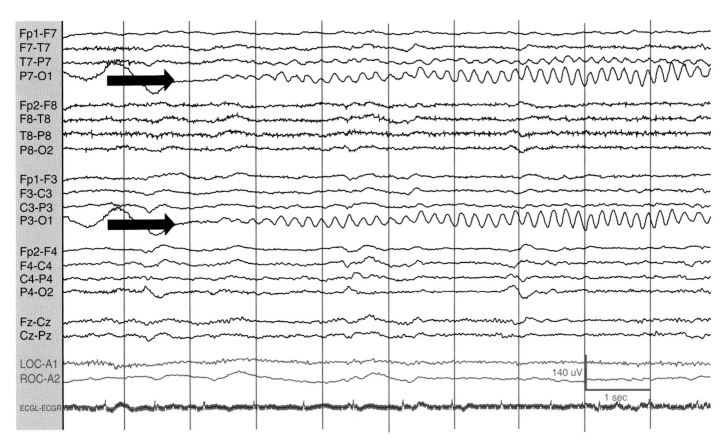

Figure 1-29 Tremor artifact. 4–6 Hz tremor artifact (arrows) posteriorly in this 66-year-old woman with Parkinson's disease. Note how there is little field anteriorly, which would be very unusual for a cerebrally generated wave.

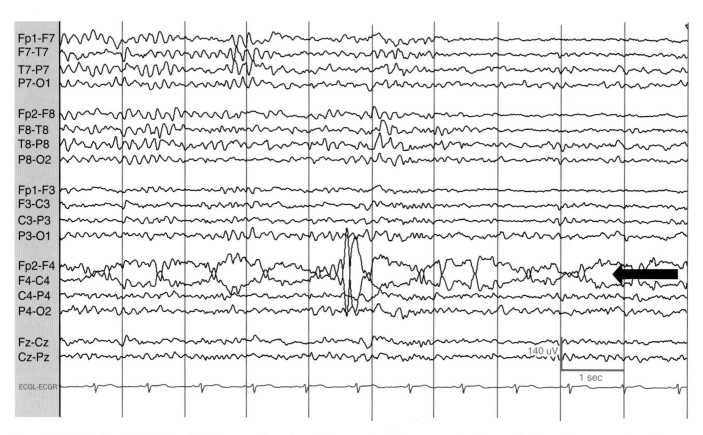

Figure 1-30 Electrode artifact. A faulty electrode contact (arrow) results in a recording with an exact mirror image referable to the common electrode (in this case, F4). In referential recording, only one channel reflects the discharge. In both cases there is no potential field. A faulty electrode can also "pop" resulting in a mirror image for only a moment.

Further reading

Adrian, E.D., Matthews, B.H.C., 1934. The Berger rhythm: potential changes from the occipital lobes in man. Brain 57, 355–385.

American Clinical Neurophysiology Society Guidelines. www.acns.org.

American, E.E.G., 1986. Society Guidelines in EEG, 1–7 (Revised 1985). J. Clin. Neurophysiol. 3, 131–168.

Andesen, P., Andersson, S.A., 1968. Physiological Basis of the Alpha Rhythm. Appleton, New York.

Beaussart, M., Guiev, J.D., Section, I.I.I., 1977. Artefacts. In: Remond, A. (Ed.), Handbook of Electroencephalography and Clinical Neurophysiology, vol. 11A. Elsevier, Amsterdam, pp. 80–96.

Berger, H., 1929. Ueber das elektroenkephalogramm des menschen. Arch Psychiatr 87, 527–570.

Binnie, C.D., 1987. Recording techniques: montages, electrodes, amplifiers and filters. In: Halliday, A.M., Butler, S.R., Paul, R. (Eds.), A Textbook of Clinical Neurophysiology. John Wiley, New York, pp. 3–22.

Binnie, C.D., Rowan, A.J., Gutter, T., 1982. A Manual of Electroencephalographic Technology. University Press, Cambridge.

Brittenham, D., 1974. Recognition and reduction of physiological artifacts. Am. J. EEG Technol. 14, 158–165.

Buzsáki, G., Anastassiou, C., Koch, C., 2012. The origin of extracellular fields and currents – EEG, ECoG, LFP and spikes. Nature Rev Neurosci 13, 407–420.

Buzsáki, G., Traub, R., Pedley, T., 2003. The Cellular Basis of EEG activity. In: Ebersole, J., Pedley, T.A. (Eds.), Current Practice of Clinical Electroencephalography. Lippincott Williams & Wilkins, Philadelphia, pp. 1–11.

Creutzfeldt, O., Houchin, J., Section, I., 1974. Neuronal basis of EEG-waves. In: Remond, A. (Ed.), Handbook of Electroencephalography and Clinical Neurophysiology, vol. 2C. Elsevier, Amsterdam, pp. 5–55.

Dempsey, E.W., Morison, R.S., 1942. The production of rhythmically recurrent cortical potentials after localized thalamic stimulation. Am. J. Physiol. 135, 293–300.

Ebersole, J.S., 2003. Cortical Generators and EEG Voltage Fields. In: Ebersole, J., Pedley, T.A. (Eds.), Current Practice of Clinical Electroencephalography. Lippincott Williams & Wilkins, Philadelphia, pp. 12–31.

Ebner, A., Sciarretta, G., Epstein, C.M., et al., 1999. EEG instrumentation. The International Federation of Clinical Neurophysiology. (Practice Guideline). Electroencephalogr. Clin. Neurophysiol. Suppl. 52, 7–10.

Goldensohn, E.S., 1979. Neurophysiological substrates of EEG activity. In: Klass, D., Daly, D. (Eds.), Current Practice of Clinical Neurophysiology. Raven, New York, pp. 421–440.

Goldman, D., 1950. The clinical use of the "average" reference electrode in monopolar recording. Electroenceph Clin Neurophysiol 2, 211–214.

Halliday, A.M., Butler, S.R., Paul, R. (Eds.), 1987. A Textbook of Clinical Neurophysiology. Wiley, Chichester, pp. 3–22.

Homan, R.W., Herman, J., Purdy, P., 1987. Cerebral localization of international 10-20 system electrode placement. Electroenceph Clin Neurophysiol 55, 376–382.

Jasper, H.H., 1958. Report of the committee on methods of clinical examination in electroencephalography. Electroenceph Clin Neurophysiol 10, 370–375.

Jasper, H.H., 1958. The ten-twenty electrode system of the International Federation. Electroenceph Clin Neurophysiol 10, 371–375.

Klass, D.W., 1977. Symposium on EEG montages: which, when, why and whither. Introduction. Am. J. EEG Technol. 17, 1–3.

Lesser, R.P., Lueders, H., Dinner, D.S., et al., 1985. An introduction to the basic concepts of polarity and localization. J. Clin. Neurophysiol. 2, 45–61.

Litt, B., Cranstoun, S.D., 2003. Engineering Principles. In: Ebersole, J., Pedley, T.A. (Eds.), Current Practice of Clinical Electroencephalography. Lippincott Williams & Wilkins, Philadelphia, pp. 32–71.

Moruzzi, G., Magoun, H.W., 1949. Brain stem reticular formation and activation of the EEG. Electroenceph Clin Neurophysiol 1, 455–473.

Saunders, M.F., 1979. Artifacts: activity of noncerebral origin in the EEG. In: Klass, D.W., Daly, D.D. (Eds.), Current Practice of Clinical Electroencephalography. Raven Press, New York, pp. 37–68.

Silverman, D., 1960. The anterior temporal electrode and the ten-twenty system. Electroenceph Clin Neurophysiol 12, 735–737.

Stones, E.A., Whitehead, M.K., MacGillivray, B.B., 1967. The nature of the eye blink artefact. Proc Electrophysiol Technol Assoc 14, 208–214.

Westmoreland, B.F., Espinosa, R.E., Klass, D.W., 1973. Significant prosopo-glossopharyngeal movements affecting the electroencephalogram. Am. J. EEG Technol. 13, 59–70.

The normal adult EEG 2

THE NORMAL EEG

Understanding the elements of the normal EEG is a prerequisite for developing expertise in interpreting the abnormal record. In the following discussion, the frequency bands and individual waveforms found in the normal adult EEG are described for both the waking and sleeping states.

ALPHA ACTIVITY

Hans Berger, the Berlin psychiatrist who in 1929 recorded the first EEG in humans, described a rhythm in the alpha frequency (8 to <13 Hz) in the posterior regions of the head. This is the posterior dominant rhythm (PDR) (Figure 2-1). The PDR is of maximal amplitude in the occipital regions and attenuates with eye opening. It is best seen when the person is in the relaxed, waking state with eyes closed. Note that waves in the alpha frequency may be found in various locations and in various states (e.g., alpha coma or during a seizure). Such waves are not the PDR as described earlier.

The PDR is in the alpha frequency in a normal adult. However, it may be slower in children or in the presence of diffuse disease processes.

In normal adults, the PDR should be above 8.5 Hz, as the PDR of 8 Hz is only seen in <1% of normal adults at any age.

In assessing the PDR, look for the patient's best – that is, the highest posterior frequency achieved during the most alert state. Slower posterior rhythms in the theta range or theta waves admixed with the alpha may be due to mild drowsiness and thus have no pathological significance.

The PDR is usually symmetric but may be of higher amplitude over the non-dominant hemisphere. In that case a 2:1 ratio is acceptable. If greater than 2:1, it may be related to an abnormality, but it also could be the result of incorrect electrode placement. The latter is more likely if the lower-amplitude alpha is well organized and equally persistent as that on the opposite side. Consideration should be given to the possible presence of an insulating process between the scalp electrodes and the cerebral cortex, as might be seen with a subdural collection. In that case the alpha on the affected side may either be markedly depressed in amplitude, or absent.

The PDR, while usually maximal in the occipital regions, often distributes to the adjacent parietal and posterior temporal areas. Moreover, this may be variable over the course of the recording.

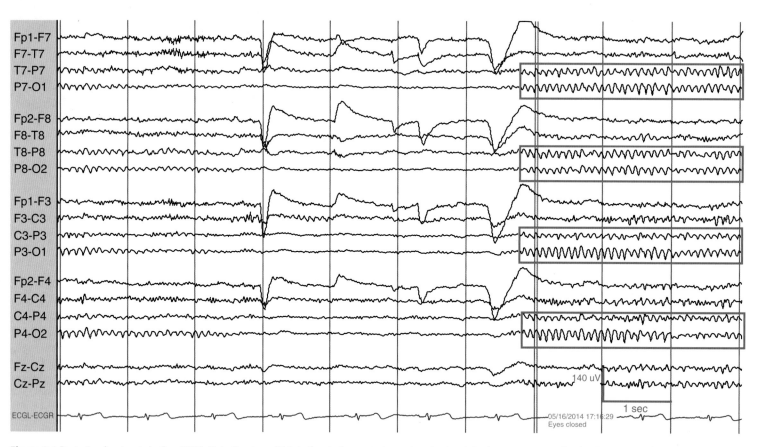

Figure 2-1 Posterior dominant rhythm (PDR). Note the sinusoidal rhythm in the posterior regions in the alpha frequency range (box). It is attenuated with eye opening and best seen with eye closure.

If the PDR increases in frequency when the patient opens his or her eyes and persists with the eyes open, or appears only during eye-opening, drowsiness is a likely cause. When the frequency transiently increases immediately after eye closure, it is called alpha squeak. Some people have little or no PDR during the resting state. This finding has no clinical significance and occurs in perhaps 5% of individuals. If the patient is tense, the PDR may not be recorded. In such cases, the PDR may appear as the patient becomes more relaxed.

Take note of processes that may lead to a decline in PDR frequency. These include (but are not limited to) effect of medication(s) such as phenytoin or valproic acid, early dementias, increased intracranial pressure, hypothyroidism, and other metabolic disorders such as hepatic insufficiency.

The absence of the PDR on one side is always pathological. In older subjects this asymmetry is often due to remote infarction. In younger subjects the cause is more likely to be brain damage such as congenital hemiatrophy. If a record contains alpha frequency and looks relatively normal, save for the fact that the alpha frequency is equally prominent in the frontal regions, interpretation depends on the state of the patient and the presence of reactivity. In a comatose patient (e.g., after cardiopulmonary arrest), with widespread alpha activity that does not react to eye movements or undergo state change, it is termed alpha coma and carries a poor prognosis.

BETA ACTIVITY

Beta activity is defined as a frequency of 13–30 Hz and is present in the background of most subjects. If completely absent it may represent an abnormality depending on other features of the EEG. Maximal beta amplitude is usually in the frontocentral regions, but it may be widespread. It does not respond to eye opening, as does the PDR. During drowsiness, beta may seem to increase in amplitude. This appears to be a function of amplitude diminution of other background frequencies and thus is more apparent than real.

Beta activity increases in amplitude and abundance by various drugs (e.g., barbiturates, chloral hydrate, benzodiazepines, and tricyclic antidepressants). In these circumstances, the beta activity is usually between 14–16 Hz (Figure 2-2).

Perhaps the most important finding when analyzing beta activity is interhemispheric asymmetry. In particular, the side of reduced amplitude usually points to the pathological hemisphere. Examples include acute and remote infarct, subdural collections, and porencephaly. By the same token, beta amplitude may be unilaterally increased. This occurs in the setting of a previous craniotomy (so-called breach artifact). In this case breach refers to an opening or rift (i.e., "Captain, there is a breach in the hull" versus "doctor, the baby is breech.") Lower impedances from the lack of skull continuity result in higher amplitudes of beta activity. Brain abscess, stroke, tumors, vascular malformations, and cortical dysplasia can be associated with either a focal decrease or an enhancement of beta activity. Beta asymmetry, if present, should always be considered in concert with asymmetry of other background frequencies.

THETA ACTIVITY

Theta activity (4–8 Hz) is often present in the waking adult EEG, although it may be completely absent. It tends to be somewhat more evident in the midline and temporal derivations. Approximately 35% of normal young adults show intermittent theta rhythm during relaxed wakefulness that is maximal in the frontocentral head regions. Also, intermittent theta frequency in temporal leads, either bilateral or unilateral (usually left more than right), can be seen in the asymptomatic elderly population with an incidence of about 35%.

If theta activity is consistently found in only one location, or is predominant over one hemisphere, it is likely to reflect underlying structural

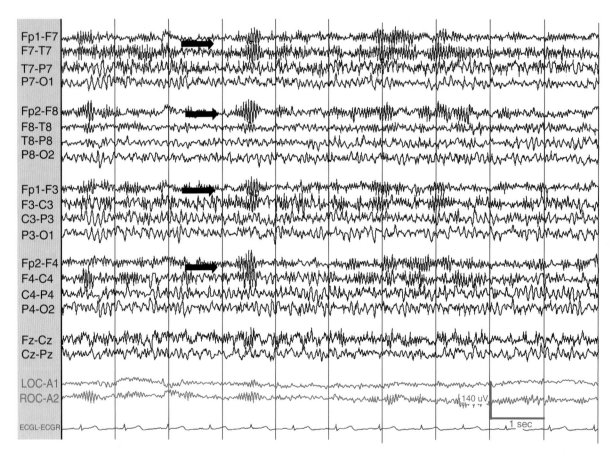

Figure 2-2 Excessive beta activity. This is a 30-year-old male on clonazepam for anxiety. The beta activity is best seen over the frontal electrodes (arrows).

disease. The lesion, however, is usually less malignant, or extensive, than in the case of delta-range focality. Examples are meningioma, low-grade glioma, and remote infarction.

Diffuse theta is usual in children. In the young, theta abundance is quite variable, and one should be flexible when determining whether the theta is excessive or not. When in doubt, err on the side of normality. In comatose patients who have suffered catastrophic brain damage, rhythmic theta may be found diffusely. This finding is termed theta coma.

DELTA ACTIVITY

Delta activity (<4 Hz) was described in 1936 by W. Gray Walter, a young English physiologist. He gathered his bulky EEG apparatus in an operating room where a patient was undergoing neurosurgery for a malignant tumor. Electrodes placed over the involved area recorded very slow, high-voltage potentials that were slower in frequency than previously reported waveforms. Walter termed these potentials delta waves. Since that time, focal delta activity has proved a reliable indicator of localized disease of the brain.

As a rule, delta waves are not present in the adult during wakefulness. It follows that their presence in wake implies cerebral dysfunction. Delta waves are a normal and important component of adult sleep.

There are other circumstances wherein delta is a normal component of the EEG. For instance, delta is prominent in infants and young children and is common in adolescents in the posterior head regions (posterior slow waves of youth).

Excessive diffuse delta is abnormal and indicates encephalopathy of non-specific etiology. Focal polymorphic delta activity usually indicates a structural lesion involving the white matter, especially when it is continuously seen. Focal rhythmic delta activity can involve the ipsilateral gray matter and be indicative of underlying cerebral hyperexcitability.

FEATURES OF SLEEP

The recording of sleep is one of the most powerful diagnostic adjuncts in electroencephalography. Relatively minor abnormalities on the routine EEG may be amplified during sleep, and new abnormalities may appear. This is particularly the case with epileptiform activity. Most patients become drowsy at some point during a routine recording, and many actually sleep spontaneously for variable periods. Focal spike or sharp wave discharges often appear or are increased during stage I (drowsiness) and stage II sleep.

Likewise, focal slow wave abnormalities may be exaggerated during these stages. With deeper sleep (slow-wave sleep, SWS) there is a tendency for epileptiform activity and focal slowing to become less obvious.

Stage I sleep is characterized by slowing, fragmentation (increasing irregularity), and ultimate disappearance of the PDR. The background may appear to be generally of lower voltage (due to absence of the PDR), and beta activity may be more obvious. Diffuse theta activity appears and increases in abundance. Vertex waves, which appear during stage I sleep, are synchronous, episodic, sharply contoured potentials (<200 ms in duration) that are maximal over the central regions. They may assume a very sharp, spike-like configuration; are variable in amplitude; and sometimes occur in rhythmic runs. In addition, positive occipital sharp transients of sleep (POSTs) may be quite prominent. These potentials have the appearance of sharp waves, are electropositive at the occipital electrodes, and may be mono- or biphasic in configuration. Do not be surprised to find long rhythmic runs of POSTs that could be mistaken for an ictal discharge by the unwary (Figure 2-3). Both vertex waves and POSTs may persist into stage II sleep.

Stage II sleep arrives with the appearance of well-defined sleep spindles and K-complexes (Figure 2-4). Sleep spindles are synchronous, sinusoidal waves at 12–14 (± 2) Hz with a potential maximum in the

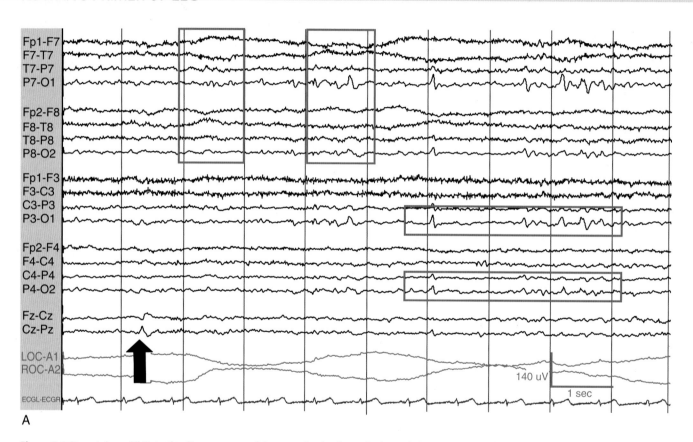

A

Figure 2-3 Stage I sleep. (A) Note the disappearance of the posterior dominant rhythm, relative attenuation of the background with more low-voltage fast activity anteriorly, slow horizontal roving eye movements (first vertical box: eyes to the left, second vertical box: eyes to the right), appearance of subtle vertex wave (arrow), and positive sharp transients of sleep (POSTs) (horizontal boxes).

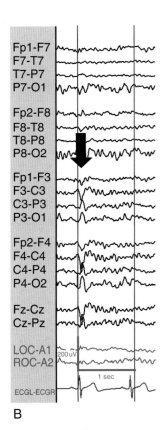

B

Figure 2-3, cont'd (B) A well-formed vertex wave (arrow) with phase reversal at the C$_z$, C$_3$, and C$_4$ electrodes.

central regions. If spindles are only fragmentary or very brief, the patient is not considered to be firmly in Stage II. K-complexes are high-voltage, synchronous bi- or triphasic slow potentials (>500 ms) usually with a central or bifrontal preponderance, often (but not invariably) in close association with sleep spindles. A K-complex can be evoked by a sudden auditory stimulus (Knock).

SWS is characterized by increasing amounts of diffuse delta activity, occupying variable amounts of the background (Figure 2-5). At the same time there is a progressive decline in sleep spindles – in fact, they may disappear. The delta may reach very high voltage without clinical significance. In adults, SWS is seldom encountered during routine recording.

Rapid eye movement (REM) sleep is characterized by rapid eye movements and loss of muscle tone (Figure 2-6). The EEG background consists of low-voltage theta activity, and eye channels demonstrate irregular vertical and horizontal eye movements. Epileptiform discharges are seldom present in REM sleep. Non-REM sleep and REM sleep alternate in cycles 4–6 times during normal sleep, with increasing REM sleep in the last third of the night. Recall that the first REM period usually occurs about 90 minutes after sleep onset, and patients with narcolepsy experience REM onset sleep. However, a routine EEG with REM may reflect sleep deprivation and does not necessarily mean a sleep disorder such as narcolepsy.

SPECIAL CONSIDERATIONS IN THE ELDERLY

At the outset let us stipulate that the EEG in the elderly, regardless of age, can be normal in every regard. This extends to the PDR, which may maintain a steady 10 Hz frequency throughout life. Alternatively, there may be a gradual decline in the frequency of the PDR. A specific disease process may not be evident, but the slower PDR probably reflects a degree of cerebral dysfunction (e.g., cerebral vascular disease or a

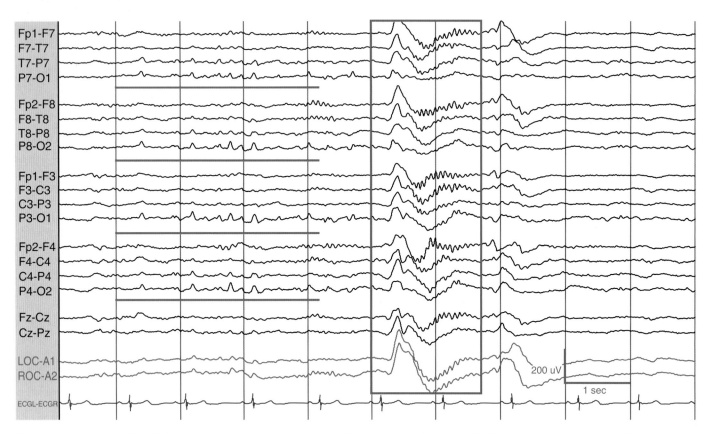

Figure 2-4 Stage II sleep. Stage II sleep is characterized by the appearance of K-complexes and sleep spindles (box). K-complexes are bifrontally or centrally predominant diffuse high-voltage, synchronous slow potentials (>500 ms). Sleep spindles often follow the K-complexes. Note runs of POSTs preceding the K-complex and spindles (underline).

46

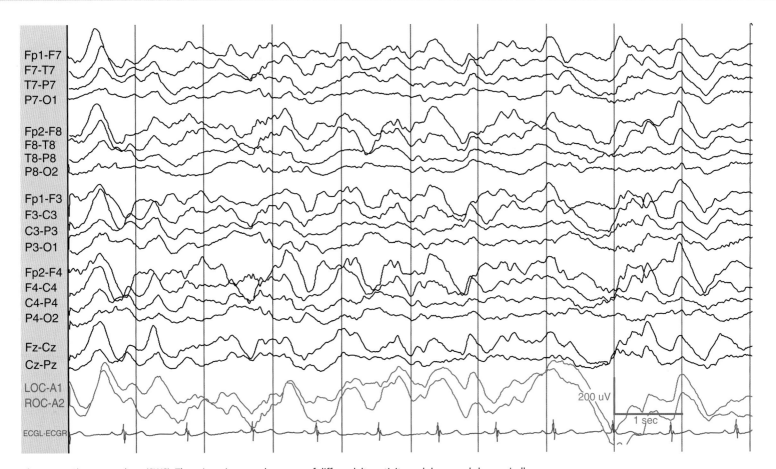

Figure 2-5 Slow wave sleep (SWS). There is an increased amount of diffuse delta activity and decreased sleep spindles.

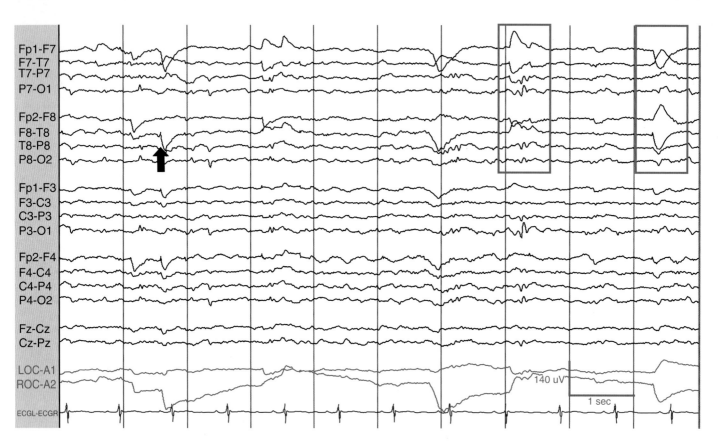

Figure 2-6 Rapid eye movement (REM) sleep. Note the irregular, fast, horizontal eye movements (first box: eyes to the left, second box: eyes to the right). They sometimes seem spiky (arrow), which represents artifacts of the lateral rectus muscles.

degenerative process). The PDR is not reported as abnormal until it falls below 8.5 Hz. Beta activity may decrease in the elderly. Another common finding is intermittent bitemporal theta and delta activity, symmetric or asymmetric, perhaps preponderant on one side. Temporal theta is generally considered normal, if it occurs in <15% of the record. Temporal delta waves probably represent underlying cerebral pathology (e.g., cerebrovascular disease). However, there may be no focal abnormality on an imaging study. We emphasize this because the ordering clinician should be aware that such a patient is relatively unlikely to have a brain tumor or stroke.

Generalized rhythmic delta activity (GRDA) with a frontal predominance is a normal finding in elderly drowsiness (previously referred to as sleep-onset FIRDA – frontal intermittent rhythmic delta activity). This feature may have no specific significance. It is possible that frontally predominant GRDA may represent some degree of subcortical dysfunction secondary to vascular disease or other degenerative factors. It is not, however, particularly helpful in making a specific diagnosis, and it is not necessary to call it abnormal in a report.

Sleep features in the elderly tend to be less well defined than those encountered in younger adults. Sleep spindles may be more irregular or of lower voltage. Similarly, vertex sharp waves may be less well defined. REM sleep is preserved in aging. However, the abundance of SWS diminishes with age.

ACTIVATION PROCEDURES

HYPERVENTILATION (HV)

HV is a standard procedure during routine EEG recording. It is thought that the usefulness of HV depends on vasoconstriction secondary to resultant decreased CO_2 concentration, thus inducing relative cerebral ischemia and decreased glucose utilization. Subjects may complain of lightheadedness or tingling in the extremities. Even tetany secondary to hypocalcemia may occur with particularly vigorous HV. The procedure is most effective in the young; in the elderly it has little effect.

The standard response is moderate to high-voltage, often rhythmic, delta and theta slowing with bifrontal preponderance (Figure 2-7). In the young, nearly continuous delta may be evoked. HV may bring out epileptiform discharges and focal slowing (Figure 2-8). In unmedicated children with absence epilepsy, it will provoke an absence seizure. As a rule, HV is carried out for 3 minutes with vigorous exhalation at an increased but not particularly rapid rate. Rapid HV moves little air and has correspondingly little effect. After the conclusion of HV the record should return to baseline levels in about 1 minute. If return to baseline occurs after a protracted period, it may represent an abnormality. The classic cause of a long return to baseline is hypoglycemia.

HV is often omitted in subjects over the age of 65 years due to its low yield. An elderly person's vascular system, probably due to disease, is less responsive to the metabolic changes precipitated by HV. In cases of suspected epilepsy, however, HV may be useful despite these limitations. Note that there are few contraindications for performing HV. In general, it is not performed in patients with pulmonary and cardiac disease. HV may be performed in patients with brain tumors, although if the resting record reveals clear focal slowing, the procedure probably offers little additional information.

PHOTIC STIMULATION (PS)

PS is another standard procedure during routine EEG recording. The procedure is easily carried out with strobe units that flash for 5–10 seconds at frequencies typically between 1 and 35 Hz. PS evokes a rhythmic frequency in the occipital derivations termed photic driving (Figure 2-9). If the response to the flash train is 1:1 it is termed the fundamental. It is not unusual to see harmonic (twice the flash

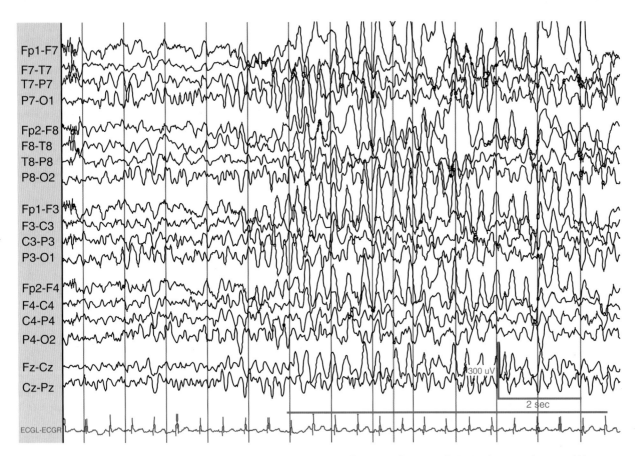

Figure 2-7 Hyperventilation. Diffuse theta and delta slowing (line) is seen with vigorous hyperventilation in this normal 7-year-old boy.

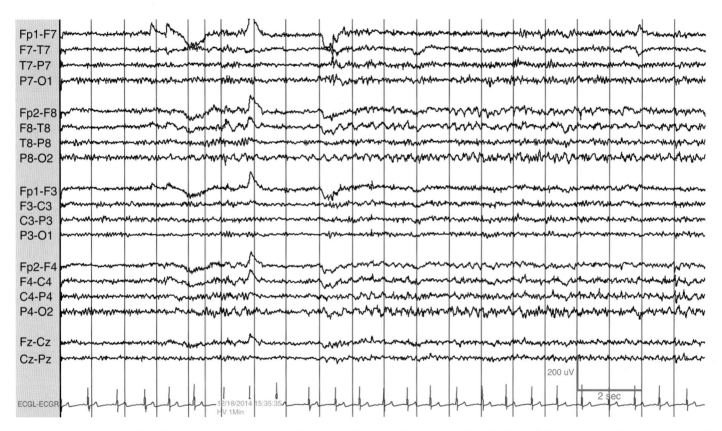

Figure 2-8 Focal slowing induced by hyperventilation: 36-year-old woman with a normal brain MRI and focal epilepsy. Right hemispheric slowing was seen with hyperventilation. The rest of the EEG showed occasional polymorphic right frontotemporal slowing.

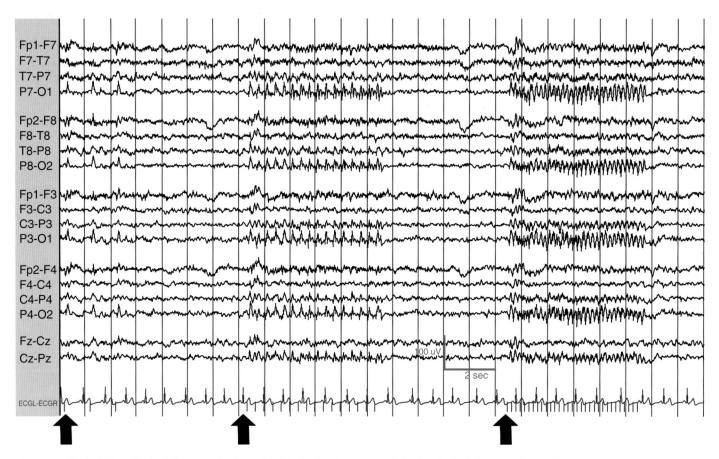

Figure 2-9 Photic driving. Rhythmic frequency in the occipital derivations is seen, time locked to the flash frequency (arrows).

frequency) and/or subharmonic (half the flash frequency) responses. Often there is no change in frequency in the occipital derivations during PS. This has no pathological significance. If photic driving is absent on one side, it may support a diagnosis of unilateral structural disease involving the occipital region (e.g., infarction in posterior cerebral artery territory). Rarely, individuals have a photomyogenic response, with myogenic potentials seen in the frontal derivations, which are time locked to the flash frequency (Figure 2-10). This is not an epileptiform abnormality!

The major utility of the procedure is in patients with epilepsy suspected of having seizures precipitated by flickering light. There are various degrees of photosensitivity, the most prominent being a synchronous high-voltage spike/polyspike wave discharge. This phenomenon is called the photoparoxysmal response (Figure 2-11). Photosensitivity is often maximal at 14–16 flashes per second. Some patients demonstrate a photoparoxysmal response at a specific frequency, or a very narrow frequency band. For patients with a marked degree of photosensitivity, an abnormal response may be obtained over a wide frequency range. Note that the technician must stop the flash train if generalized polyspike-wave bursts occur. If the stimulus is continued, a generalized convulsion may result. Typically, the evoked discharges outlast cessation of the flash stimulus by a second or so.

SLEEP DEPRIVATION

Sleep deprivation is a powerful activator of epileptiform activity. It is sometimes suggested that the subject stay up all night before his or her appointment the next morning, but a brief period of sleep may be permitted. In the latter case the patient is instructed to stay up late, sleep for 1 or 2 hours, and then come to the EEG laboratory for testing in the morning. No caffeinated beverages are permitted, as the goal is to have the patient sleep for a portion of the recording. Hyperventilation

is carried out early in the test, after which the patient is allowed to sleep. One can expect an increase in or de novo appearance of focal epileptiform activity in about 30% of patients with epilepsy. Sleep deprivation is often used during a video EEG admission in order to increase the probability of capturing the patient's typical seizure.

NORMAL VARIANTS AND PAROXYSMAL PHENOMENA OF UNCERTAIN SIGNIFICANCE

Alpha variants

Slow alpha variant appears in the occipital regions at a frequency one-half that of the ongoing PDR. Suspect its presence when PDR activity has a notched appearance, revealing its subharmonic relationship. Slow alpha variant has the same characteristics as the PDR itself – for example, it attenuates with eye opening. Fast alpha variant also appears in the occipital areas and has a frequency twice that of the PDR (Figure 2-12). These variants may alternate with the PDR, or the PDR may not be present at all. Both are normal.

Mu rhythm

Mu rhythm is normal, found in the central derivations (C3/C4) over the motor strip (Figure 2-13). It may be unilateral or bilateral; if bilateral it may be synchronous or asynchronous. Mu is sometimes more evident during drowsiness and when the eyes are open. It is considered to be related to beta activity, possibly a subharmonic. Mu attenuates with movement of the opposite upper limb (e.g., making a fist), or even thinking about such an action. It is often prominent over the site of a craniotomy. The importance of mu lies mainly in its recognition as a normal finding.

Lambda waves

Lambda waves are electropositive transients recorded in the occipital regions (Figure 2-14). They are sharply contoured, usually symmetric,

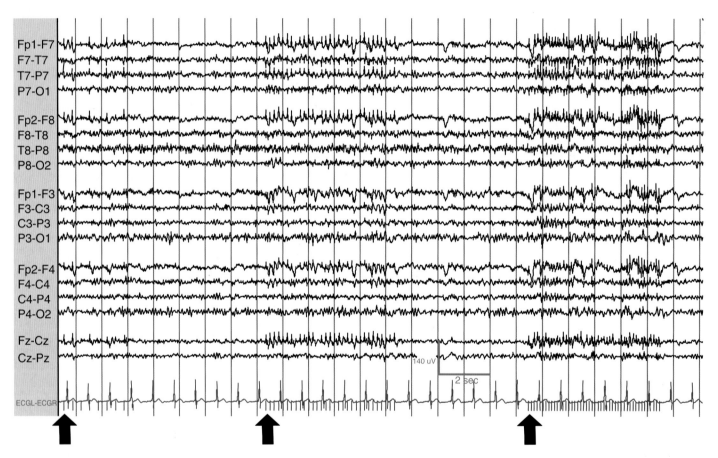

Figure 2-10 Photomyogenic response: Myogenic potentials (EMG artifacts) are seen in the frontal derivations, time locked to the flash frequency (arrows).

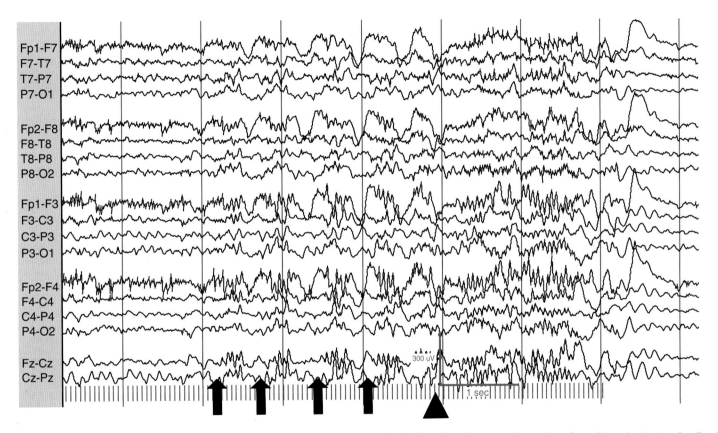

Figure 2-11 Photoparoxysmal response. At 17 Hz photic stimulation, this 18-year-old girl with reflex epilepsy gets intermittent frontally predominant polyspikes (arrows) followed by a two second run of polyspikes (arrowhead). She typically finds this pleasurable (at home will self-induce in front of the TV) and is not compliant with medication.

55

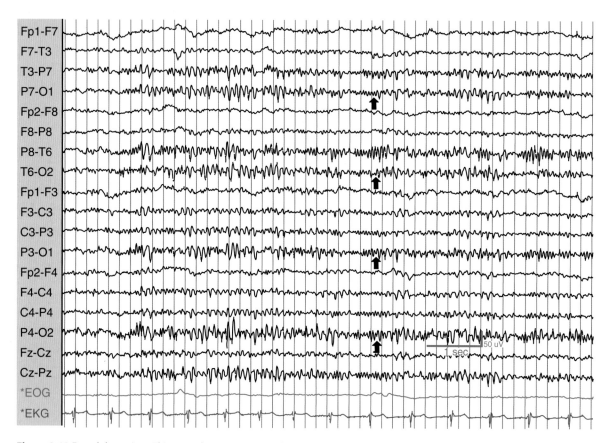

Figure 2-12 Fast alpha variant. This normal variant consists of a rapid frequency that is twice the normal PDR. In this case the variant is prominent in the posterior quadrants at a frequency of 20 Hz. It has the same general characteristics as the alpha (e.g., attenuation with eye opening).

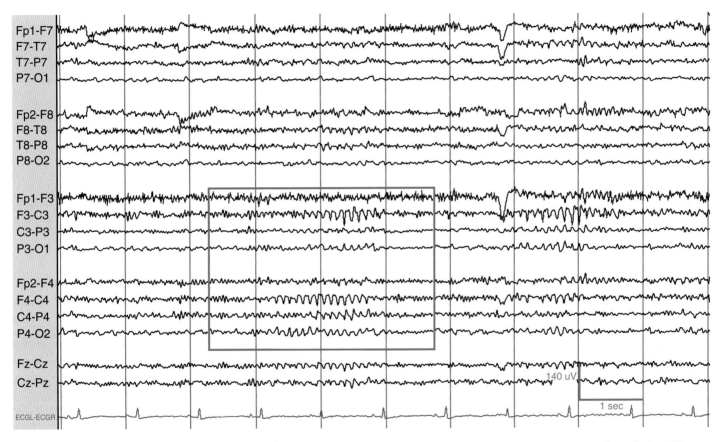

Figure 2-13 Mu rhythm. Mu rhythm consists of arch-shaped centrally predominant waves (rectangle) at 7–11 Hz. When the arm is moved, mu rhythm will attenuate contralateral to the movement. In fact, if the subject even thinks about moving an arm (say the right arm), mu rhythm will attenuate on the left.

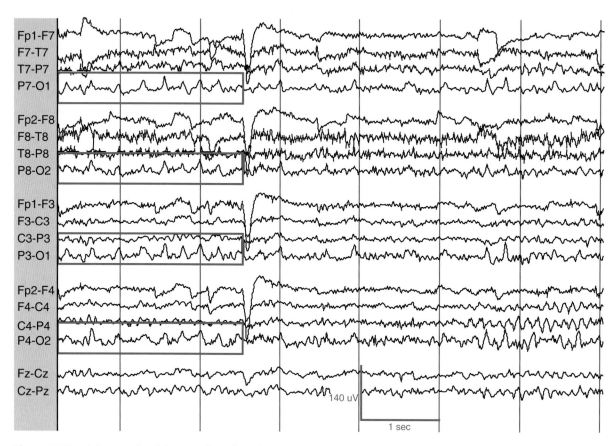

Figure 2-14 Lambda waves. Lambda waves (boxes) are sharp transients of positive polarity, recorded in the occipital region (positive at 01/02; negative at P7/P8/P3/P4) induced in the waking state by scanning the environment.

and can be mistaken for epileptiform potentials. At the same time, lambda often goes unnoticed due to lack of awareness by the reader, as well as the absence of circumstances, which lead to their expression, namely scanning eye movements. Having the subject look at a picture containing interesting subjects or details may provoke lambda waves. Lambda waves probably represent visual evoked potentials. Again, the principal advantage to recognizing lambda is the knowledge that it is a normal finding and not an example of epileptiform activity.

Rhythmic mid-temporal theta discharges (RMTD)

This was formerly known as psychomotor variant. RMTD consists of rhythmic sharply contoured theta waves at 5–6 Hz in the midtemporal regions (Figure 2-15). The bursts are brief, usually 1 sec or so in duration, and may be unilateral or independent in both midtemporal regions. This phenomenon appears during drowsiness and has no clear clinical significance. Incidentally, psychomotor variant (the old term) was meant to suggest that this phenomenon might be correlated with complex partial seizures (formerly psychomotor seizures). In fact, this usually does not turn out to be the case. Nonetheless, RMTD is sometimes considered an abnormality by the inexperienced.

Wicket spikes

Wicket spikes are sharply contoured rhythmic frequencies varying from 7–11 Hz, maximal in the midtemporal derivations, occurring in brief runs (Figure 2-16). Wicket spikes look like a comb or wicket fence. At times, one of the waves may stand out from the others, giving the appearance of a sharp wave or a spike. Noting the durations of the waveforms to be similar, regardless of variations in amplitude, makes the diagnosis. Unlike epileptiform sharp waves or spikes, there is no aftergoing slow wave. This finding occurs during drowsiness and has no apparent clinical significance. The reader should compare the locations of wicket spikes and mu rhythm (the latter is found in the central regions).

Subclinical rhythmic electroencephalographic discharges of adults (SREDA)

SREDA masquerades as an electrographic seizure in one or both hemispheres (Figure 2-17). Unlike most other benign variants that occur more in young adults in a drowsy state, this pattern typically occurs in the older population (over 50 years of age) and is seen in wake and sleep. It is typically maximal at the temporoparietal junction but can be seen at the vertex as well. It may appear in two forms: (1) symmetric or asymmetric bilateral bursts of rhythmic sharply contoured theta activity; or (2) sudden appearance of repetitive sharp or slow waveforms that become shorter in interval followed by a sustained burst that mimics the evolution of an electrographic seizure. SREDA usually lasts 40–80 seconds, and during this time the patient has no alteration of awareness and is fully responsive. SREDA has no known significance beyond the fact that it must be recognized in order to avoid misdiagnosis.

Small sharp spikes (SSS)

SSSs are low-amplitude, rapid spikes (Figure 2-18). They appear in both hemispheres as synchronous or asynchronous, most often in the temporal derivations, and become evident during drowsiness and light sleep. They are not thought to be associated with epilepsy. Small sharp spikes are also known as benign epileptiform transients of sleep (BETS).

Phantom spike-wave discharges

Phantom spike-waves are usually synchronous discharges at a frequency of 5–6 Hz appearing symmetrically (Figure 2-19). They can have either an anterior or a posterior predominance. The spike itself is usually

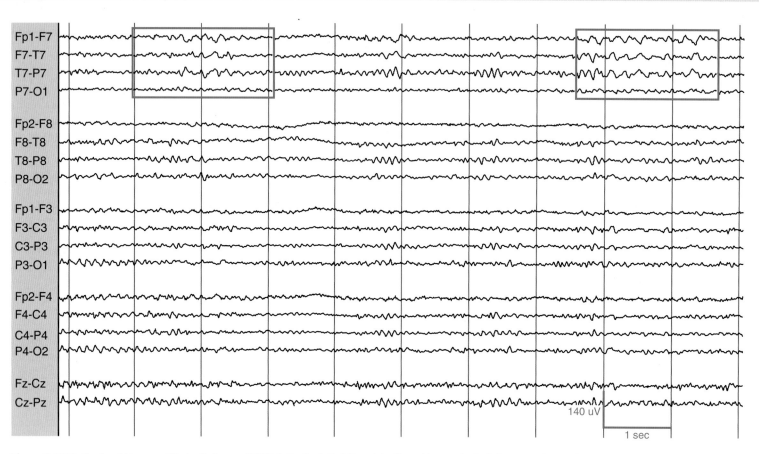

Figure 2-15 Rhythmic mid-temporal theta discharges (RMTDs). Rhythmic 5–6 Hz activity (boxes) is seen in the left temporal area of a 44-year-old woman who was hospitalized for new-onset psychogenic non-epileptic attacks. This woman had bilateral abundant RMTDs. RMTDs are a normal variant.

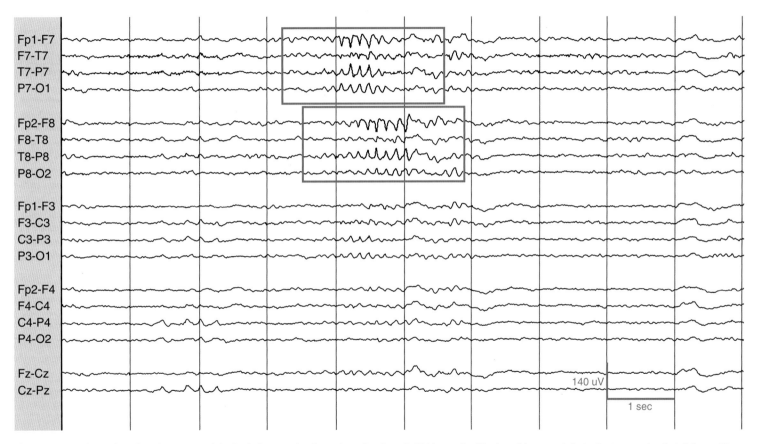

Figure 2-16 Wicket spikes. Sharply contoured rhythmic frequencies (boxes) varying from 7–11 Hz, maximal in the midtemporal derivations, occurring in brief runs. The duration of the waveforms is similar and there is no aftergoing slow wave. Wicket spikes are normal.

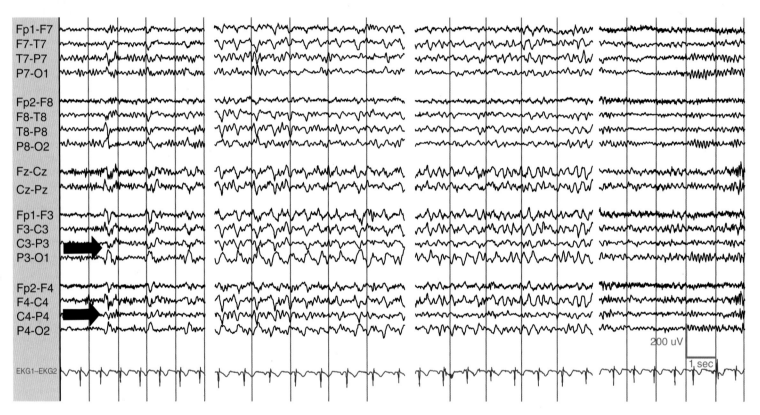

Figure 2-17 Subclinical rhythmic electroencephalographic discharge of adults (SREDA). This 58-year-old man suffered an episode of syncope, and EEGs showed multiple episodes of SREDA with sharply contoured bilateral temporoparietal delta (arrows) that became closer in interval and then resolved with no clinical correlate. He was erroneously treated with AEDs, which had no impact on the pattern. He has been off AEDs for several years and has not had any clinical episodes, though this pattern persists.

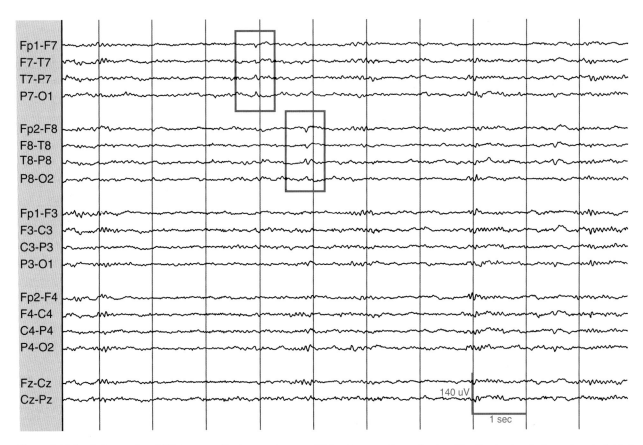

Figure 2-18 Small sharp spikes (SSS). Low-amplitude, asynchronous bilateral temporally maximal rapid spikes (rectangles) seen here in light sleep. These are not associated with epilepsy.

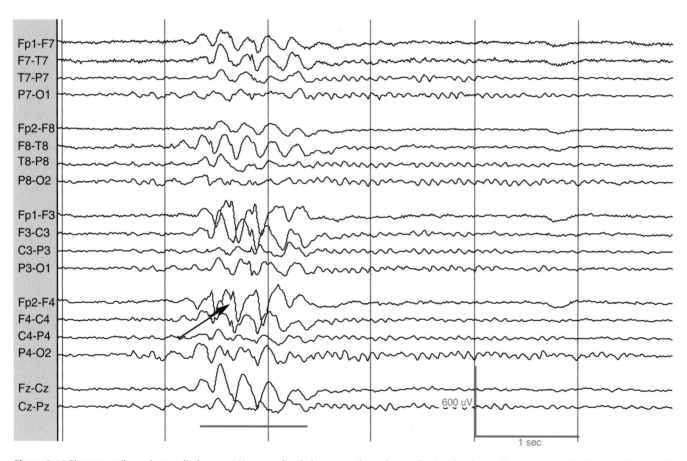

Figure 2-19 Phantom spike and wave discharges. 5 Hz generalized phantom spike and wave (line) with subtle spikes (arrow) in this 19-year-old man with psychosis.

less prominent than the following slow wave. Spikes appear individually or in brief rhythmic runs and do not have known epileptogenic significance.

14 and 6 (14/6) positive spikes

14 and 6 positive spikes, as the name implies, are positive in polarity. They are usually maximal in the posterior quadrants and appear in isolation or in groups. They may be unilateral or bilateral. The two frequencies are often admixed, but one may predominate. The phenomenon appears during drowsiness and is best recorded with crossed ear references (essentially wide interelectrode distances). In the past, 14/6 was thought to be associated with a wide variety of conditions including psychiatric disorders and epilepsy. Although there remains some disagreement as to their significance, they have no known relationship to epilepsy.

Further reading

Binnie, C.D., Coles, P.A., Margerison, J.H., 1969. The influence of end-tidal carbon dioxide tension on EEG changes during routine hyperventilation in different age groups. Electroencephalogr. Clin. Neurophysiol. 27 (3), 304–306.

Dement, W., Kleitman, N., 1957. Cyclic variations in EEG during sleep and their relation to eye movements, body motility, and dreaming. Electroencephalogr. Clin. Neurophysiol. 9 (4), 673–690.

Ellingson, R.J., Wilken, K., Bennett, D.R., 1984. Efficacy of sleep deprivation as an activation procedure in epilepsy patients. J. Clin. Neurophysiol. 1 (1), 83–101.

Erwin, C.W., Somerville, E.R., Radtke, R.A., 1984. A review of electroencephalographic features of normal sleep. J. Clin. Neurophysiol. 1 (3), 253–274.

Fountain, N.B., Kim, J.S., Lee, S.I., 1998. Sleep deprivation activates epileptiform discharges independent of the activating effects of sleep. J. Clin. Neurophysiol. 15 (1), 69–75.

Gabor, A.J., Seyal, M., 1986. Effect of sleep on the electrographic manifestations of epilepsy. J. Clin. Neurophysiol. 3 (1), 23–38.

Gloor, P., Tsai, C., Haddad, F., 1958. An assessment of the value of sleep-electroencephalography for the diagnosis of temporal lobe epilepsy. Electroencephalogr. Clin. Neurophysiol. 10 (4), 633–648.

Hartikainen, P., Soininen, H., Partanen, J., et al., 1992. Aging and spectral analysis of EEG in normal subjects: a link to memory and CSF AChE. Acta. Neurol. Scand. 86, 148–155.

Heppenstall, M.E., 1944. The relation between the effects of the blood sugar levels and hyperventilation on the electroencephalogram. J. Neurol. Neurosurg. Psychiatr. 7 (3–4), 112–118.

Hubbard, O., Sunde, D., 1976. Goldensohn ES. The EEG in centenarians. Electroencephalogr. Clin. Neurophysiol. 40 (4), 407–417.

Hughes, J.R., 1960. Usefulness of photic stimulation in routine clinical electroencephalography. Neurology 10, 777–782.

Hughes, J.R., 1977. Cayaffa JJ. The EEG in patients at different ages without organic cerebral disease. Electroencephalogr. Clin. Neurophysiol. 42 (6), 776–784.

Klass, D.W., Brenner, R.P., 1995. Electroencephalography of the elderly. J. Clin. Neurophysiol. 12 (2), 116–131.

Klass, D.W., Westmoreland, B.F., 1985. Nonepileptogenic epileptiform electroencephalographic activity. Ann. Neurol. 18 (6), 627–635.

Kozelka, J.W., Pedley, T.A., 1990. Beta and mu rhythms. J. Clin. Neurophysiol. 7 (2), 191–207.

Lipman, I.J., Hughes, J.R., 1969. Rhythmic mid-temporal discharges. An electro-clinical study. Electroencephalogr. Clin. Neurophysiol. 27 (1), 43–47.

Markand, O.N., 1990. Alpha rhythms. J. Clin. Neurophysiol. 7 (2), 163–189.

O'Brien, T.J., Sharbrough, F.W., Westmoreland, B.F., et al., 1998. Subclinical rhythmic electrographic discharges of adults (SREDA) revisited: a study using digital EEG analysis. J. Clin. Neurophysiol. 15 (6), 493–501.

Patel, V.M., Maulsby, R.L., 1987. How hyperventilation alters the electroencephalogram: a review of controversial viewpoints emphasizing neurophysiological mechanisms. J. Clin. Neurophysiol. 4 (2), 101–120.

Pratt, K.L., Mattson, R.H., Weikers, N.J., et al., 1968. EEG activation of epileptics following sleep deprivation: a prospective study of 114 cases. Electroencephalogr. Clin. Neurophysiol. 24 (1), 11–15.

Reiher, J., Lebel, M., 1977. Wicket spikes: clinical correlates of a previously undescribed EEG pattern. Can. J. Neurol. Sci. 4 (1), 39–47.

Reilly, E.L., Peters, J.F., 1973. Relationship of some varieties of electroencephalographic photosensitivity to clinical convulsive disorders. Neurology 23 (10), 1050–1057.

Rowan, A.J., Siegel, M., Rosenbaum, D.H., 1987. Daytime intensive monitoring: comparison with prolonged intensive and ambulatory monitoring. Neurology 37 (3), 481–484.

Rowan, A.J., Veldhuisen, R.J., Nagelkerke, N.J., 1982. Comparative evaluation of sleep deprivation and sedated sleep EEGs as diagnostic aids in epilepsy. Electroencephalogr. Clin. Neurophysiol. 54 (4), 357–364.

Tatum, W.O., 2013. Normal "suspicious" EEG. Neurology 80 (1 Suppl. 1), S4–S11.

Tatum, WOt, Husain, A.M., Benbadis, S.R., et al., 2006. Normal adult EEG and patterns of uncertain significance. J. Clin. Neurophysiol. 23 (3), 194–207.

Thomas, J.E., Klass, D.W., 1968. Six-per-second spike-and-wave pattern in the electroencephalogram. A reappraisal of its clinical significance. Neurology 18 (6), 587–593.

Veldhuizen, R., Binnie, C.D., Beintema, D.J., 1983. The effect of sleep deprivation on the EEG in epilepsy. Electroencephalogr. Clin. Neurophysiol. 55 (5), 505–512.

Visser, S.L., Hooijer, C., Jonker, C., et al., 1987. Anterior temporal focal abnormalities in EEG in normal aged subjects; correlations with psychopathological and CT brain scan findings. Electroencephalogr. Clin. Neurophysiol. 66 (1), 1–7.

Westmoreland, B.F., Klass, D.W., 1986. Midline theta rhythm. Arch. Neurol. 43 (2), 139–141.

Westmoreland, B.F., Klass, D.W., 1997. Unusual variants of subclinical rhythmic electrographic discharge of adults (SREDA). Electroencephalogr. Clin. Neurophysiol. 102 (1), 1–4.

Westmoreland, B.F., Reiher, J., Klass, D.W., 1979. Recording small sharp spikes with depth electroencephalography. Epilepsia 20 (6), 599–606.

White, J.C., Langston, J.W., Pedley, T.A., 1977. Benign epileptiform transients of sleep. Clarification of the small sharp spike controversy. Neurology 27 (11), 1061–1068.

The normal EEG from neonates to adolescents 3

NEONATES

Neonatal EEGs are perhaps the most challenging for the student and even for the experienced electroencephalographer. In the neonatal period, the brain is developing rapidly. Within the first 24 weeks of gestation, the cortical layers of the brain form with migration of neurons and glial cells from the periventricular germinal zone to the cortex. From 24 weeks to term, the brain goes from having a smooth surface to having the intricate pattern of sulcation characteristic of the adult brain. Myelination occurs almost exclusively after birth. Not surprisingly, these changes all impact the neonatal EEG.

For this reason, it is imperative that the electroencephalographer know the conceptual age (CA) of the neonate. The CA is the sum of the gestation age (GA – the number of weeks since the last menstrual cycle) and the legal age (age since time of birth). Term newborns are born at 37–44 weeks GA, preterm newborns <37 weeks GA, and post-term newborns >44 weeks GA. What is normal for a 26-week-old premature infant represents severe cerebral dysfunction for a full-term infant. Persistence or reappearance of a premature pattern for the CA is a sign of dysmaturity or cerebral dysfunction.

In addition, the neonatal study ideally includes several polygraphic recordings to help ascertain the behavioral state of the neonate, as well as to assess for apnea. These include electrodes to measure eye movements and muscle tone (with a submental or chin electrode) and transducers to measure airflow (a nasal thermistor) and respiratory effort (a thoracic strain gauge). As with adults, in central apnea, there is no activity in either the thoracic strain gauge or nasal thermistor. There is no breathing in central apnea because there is no effort to breathe. In contrast, with obstructive apnea, there is no flow in the nasal thermistor as air is not able to enter, but there is effort in the thoracic strain gauge.

Neonatal EEG recordings may be performed with a full number of electrodes in the usual 10-10 formation. Alternatively, due to the small head size of the neonate, a reduced array can be used. The neonatal EEG is typically read with a speed of 15 mm/second. This is contrasted with the adult speed of 30 mm/second. This compresses the data of the neonate and facilitates evaluation of continuity and symmetry.

As with all complex analyses, we recommend a systematic approach to the evaluation of the neonatal EEG. Specifically, continuity, symmetry, EEG features, sleep/wake cycle, and reactivity should be examined for each neonatal EEG (see Table 3-1).

Table 3-1 Conceptual age and the EEG

Conceptual age	Continuity	Synchrony	EEG features	Sleep/wake cycles	Reactivity
24–29 weeks	**Tracé discontinu:** EEG may be entirely flat.	90–100%	**Delta brush:** Located frequently over the central and midline areas. **Monorhythmic occipital delta activity:** Runs last only a few seconds. **Theta bursts:** Appear at 26 weeks.	**No sleep/wake cycles:** Respiration always irregular.	**Not reactive**
29–32 weeks	**Tracé discontinu:** IBI 6–35 seconds. **Continuous activity:** Rare but may be seen in wake and active sleep.	50–70%	**Delta brush:** More abundant; more prominent in active sleep. **Monorhythmic occipital delta activity:** Runs can last more than 30 seconds. **Theta bursts:** Maximal at this CA.	**Awake/active sleep:** EEG is continuous. REM seen in active sleep. **Quiet sleep:** Tracé discontinu. **Indeterminate:** Majority of EEG is indeterminate.	**Not reactive**
32–35 weeks	**Tracé discontinu:** IBI become fewer and briefer (<10 seconds). **Continuous activity:** May be seen in wake and active sleep.		**Delta brushes:** Most frequent over temporal and occipital regions. More common in quiet sleep. **Monorhythmic occipital delta activity:** Fading in occipital regions. **Theta bursts:** Cease. **Multifocal sharp transients:** Maximal at this CA.	**Awake/active sleep:** EEG is continuous. **Quiet sleep:** Tracé discontinu. **Indeterminate:** Much of the EEG is still indeterminate.	**Reactive**
35–37 weeks	**Tracé alternant:** Relative discontinuity between 4 and 6 seconds. Seen in quiet sleep. **Continuous activity:** In wake and active sleep.	60–85%	**Delta brushes:** More frequent during quiet sleep. **Multifocal sharp transients:** Less abundant. **Frontal sharp waves (encoches frontales):** Maximally expressed at this CA. **Monorhythmic frontal delta**	**Awake:** Activité moyenne pattern dominates. **Active sleep:** REM, decreased EMG, activité moyenne predominates on EEG. **Quiet sleep:** Respirations more regular, tracé alternant pattern on EEG.	**Reactive**

Table 3-1 continued

Conceptual age	Continuity	Synchrony	EEG features	Sleep/wake cycles	Reactivity
37–44 weeks	**Tracé alternant:** Can be seen in quiet sleep. **Continuous activity:** Majority of record is continuous except quiet sleep, which can show a tracé alternant pattern.	90–100%	**Delta brushes:** Very infrequent. **Multifocal sharp transients:** Typically resolve. **Frontal sharp waves (encoches frontales):** Diminish by 44 weeks CA.	**Awake:** Activité moyenne or mixed pattern. **Active sleep:** REM, decreased EMG, activité moyenne predominates on EEG. **Quiet sleep:** Respirations more regular, tracé alternant pattern or continuous slow wave pattern.	**Reactive**

CONTINUITY

The normal EEG evolution is one of persistent discontinuity in the premature infant to one of continuity in a fully mature infant. A premature infant of less than 29 weeks CA may have an EEG that is entirely flat or flat with medium to high amplitude bursts (50–300 µV). Between 29–32 weeks CA, the interburst interval (IBI) is typically 6–8 seconds but can be as long as 35 seconds. The amplitude of the IBI is less than 25 µV. This pattern is known as tracé discontinu (Figure 3-1). Rare periods of continuous activity may be seen in wake and active sleep. Between 32 and 35 weeks CA the IBI becomes shorter and is rarely greater than 10 seconds. At this time continuous activity may be seen in wake and in active sleep. At 35 weeks CA the tracé discontinu is shifting into a less discontinuous pattern called tracé alternant (Figure 3-2). In tracé alternant, the periods of relative discontinuity are shorter (typically 4–6 seconds) and higher in amplitude (>25 µV). The EEG shows a tracé alternant pattern in quiet sleep and continuous activity in wake and active sleep. Between 37 and 44 weeks CA, the EEG should be continuous except for quiet sleep, which can maintain a tracé alternant pattern. After 44 weeks, the EEG should be continuous at all times.

INTERHEMISPHERIC SYNCHRONY

The hemispheres are defined as synchronous if there is less than a 1.5-second difference in the onset of EEG activity during a discontinuous background. The development of the neonatal EEG is interesting because synchrony is initially abundant (Figure 3-1) and then decreases and increases again. Specifically, premature infants less than 29 weeks have a high level of synchrony (90–100%). Synchrony nadirs between 31 and 32 weeks CA with approximately 50–70% of bursts being synchronous (Figure 3-3). After this, synchrony gradually increases (Figure 3-2). Between 37 and 44 weeks CA, nearly 100% of bursts (seen during quiet sleep when there is a tracé alternant pattern) are synchronous.

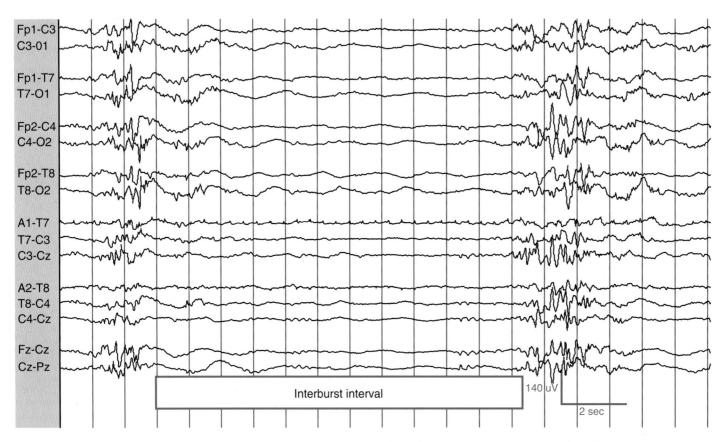

Figure 3-1 Tracé discontinu, synchronous. Tracé discontinu pattern seen in a 29.5-week CA infant. Interburst interval is 9 seconds and bursts are synchronous. Note subtle EKG artifact in A1-T7 channel.

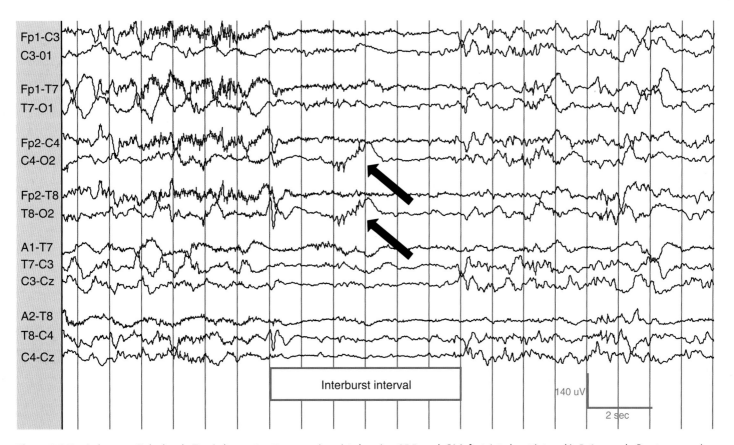

Figure 3-2 Tracé alternant. Delta brush. Tracé alternant pattern seen in quiet sleep in a 35.5-week CA infant. Interburst interval is 5–6 seconds. Bursts are synchronous. Arrows point to right occipital delta brush.

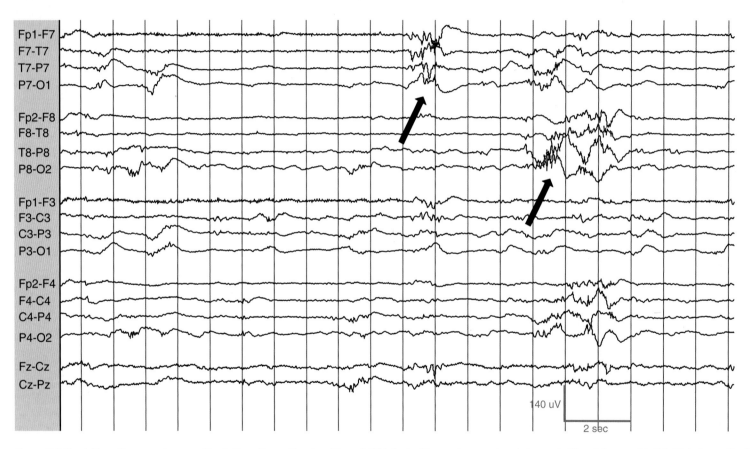

Figure 3-3 Tracé discontinu, asynchronous. Tracé discontinu pattern in a 31-week CA infant with asynchronous bursts (separated by >1.5 seconds). This CA is the nadir of synchrony.

EEG FEATURES

At different neonatal ages, there is the development of certain characteristic waveforms. These are either not seen at all in adult life (delta brush) or seen in adult life but may have an entirely different significance (sharp waves/transients). The following background elements appear, peak and then fade during particular periods of neonatal development.

The first characteristic waveform to be seen is the delta brush pattern, which can be present as early as 24 weeks CA. This is a slow moderate-to high-amplitude delta wave with superimposed lower amplitude fast frequencies. Between 24 and 29 weeks CA delta brushes are seen mostly over the central and midline areas but by 32–35 weeks CA delta brushes are seen mostly in the occipital and temporal regions (Figure 3-2). Prior to 33 weeks CA, the delta brushes are seen primarily in active sleep. After 33 weeks CA, the delta brush pattern is seen primarily in quiet sleep. Delta brushes are infrequent by 37 weeks and, if abundant, should be taken as evidence of possible dysmaturity.

Monorhythmic occipital delta activity consists of runs of high amplitude posterior delta. This activity occurs symmetrically and synchronously usually in the bilateral occipital regions. It has a similar time course as delta brush, first appearing at 24 weeks CA, peaking between 31 and 33 weeks, and fading by 35 weeks. In an infant less than 29 weeks, CA monorhythmic occipital delta activity rarely lasts more than a few seconds in duration. By 31 weeks CA runs of monorhythmic occipital delta can last for more than 30 seconds. This is often admixed with delta brush.

Theta bursts, also known as temporal sawtooth waves, are seen starting at 26 weeks CA and maximal in the relatively narrow CA bandwidth of 29 to 32 weeks CA. These occur in the temporal electrodes independently for 1–2 seconds and consist of sharply contoured rhythmic theta waves, with amplitudes of up to 200 μV.

Starting at 32 weeks CA, during continuous portions of EEG, there is the development of a rarely present amplitude gradient with higher amplitudes posteriorly (in the delta range) and lower-amplitude, faster activity anteriorly. This gradient is maintained in adult life (though the frequencies are different) and becomes the cornerstone of an organized adult EEG.

Multifocal sharp transients (Figure 3-4) are most frequent between 32 and 34 weeks CA but can persist and are considered normal up to 46 weeks CA. These are sharp waves, which can be maximal in essentially any location.

After 34 weeks, frontal sharp waves (also known as encoches frontales) become more frequent as multifocal sharp transients become less frequent. Frontal sharp waves usually occur in isolation or in brief runs and are typically synchronous and symmetric (Figure 3-5). They may appear as early as 26 weeks CA but are polyphasic with high amplitudes. Typically there is a small initial negative deflection and a larger positive deflection. They diminish at 44 weeks CA, rarely seen during sleep after 46 weeks CA and disappear by 48 weeks CA. Frontal monorhythmic delta is seen around 34 weeks CA. This pattern often appears with admixed frontal sharp waves. Both multifocal sharp transients and frontal sharp waves can occur in any state. As these have a morphology similar to adult sharp waves, it is a common rookie mistake to report these as abnormal and as a marker for a possible seizure disorder. Even if these persist past 46 weeks CA, they are a more non-specific sign of cerebral dysfunction and may not be secondary to cortical hyper-excitability. If sharp waves are overly frequent at any one location, occur for long periods of time, and/or have persistent asymmetry, it is abnormal at any age.

SLEEP/WAKE CYCLE

Before 29 weeks CA, sleep wake cycles do not exist. Respirations are exclusively irregular. Between 29 and 32 weeks CA, there is the emergence of rarely identifiable quiet and active sleep. At this age, wake and active

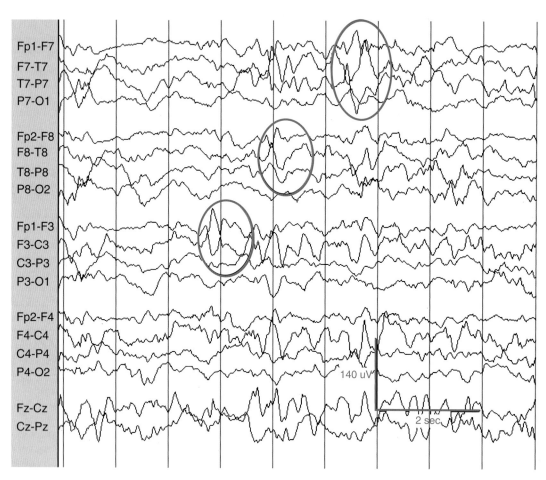

Figure 3-4 Multifocal sharp transients. Multifocal sharp transients seen in this 36-week CA infant.

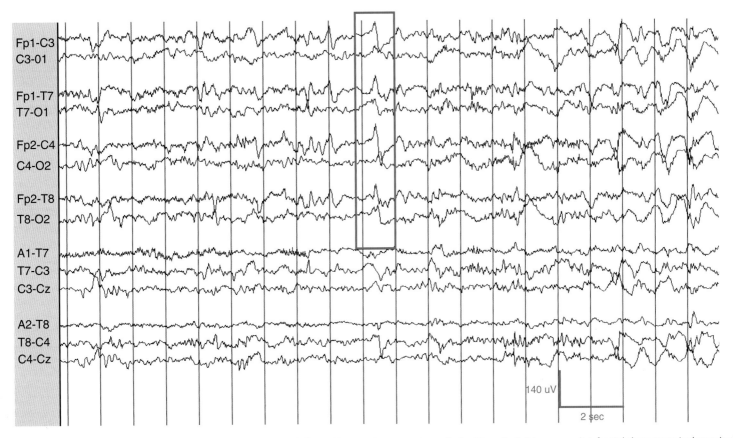

Figure 3-5 Activité moyenne. Frontal sharp wave. 39.5-week CA infant with a continuous pattern of mixed type (activité moyenne). A frontal sharp wave is shown in the box.

sleep look the same on EEG and are continuous. In active sleep, in addition to EEG continuity, there are rapid eye movements (REM), irregular respirations, and increased muscle tone in the submental EMG (chin muscle tone). In quiet sleep, respirations are regular and the EEG shows a tracé discontinu pattern. Much of sleep remains indeterminate, which means that sleep states cannot be clearly identified as quiet or active sleep.

By 35 weeks CA, there is a decrease in tonic EMG in active sleep. This is maintained throughout childhood and adult life as muscle tone is low in active sleep/REM sleep. In the pathological circumstance of REM behavior disorder in adults, this paralysis is lost, and people will act out their dreams resulting in punching, kicking, screaming, leg bicycling, and even getting out of bed. By 35 weeks CA, a mixed pattern (activité moyenne), which contains both low- and medium-amplitude components of varying frequencies, dominates the awake and active sleep record (Figure 3-5). During active sleep at this age there are more rapid eye movements during REM. Quiet sleep has longer periods of regular respirations.

By 37 weeks CA wakefulness, active and quiet sleep can be clearly delineated on the EEG. Active sleep and wakefulness consist of activité moyenne. At term, approximately 80% of sleep onset and 50% of overall sleep consists of active (REM) sleep. Quiet sleep consists of either a tracé alternant pattern or a continuous slow wave pattern, which is a more mature feature. In between waking, active sleep, and quiet sleep there is something called transitional sleep, which represents a behavioral and EEG pattern not completely fulfilling criteria for the previously mentioned patterns.

REACTIVITY

The neonatal EEG is not reactive to stimulation until 32 weeks CA. After 32 weeks CA, stimulation will cause either a widespread attenuation of

activity or, less often, an augmentation of activity on the EEG. If the baby is in quiet sleep with a tracé alternant pattern, stimulation may cause a transition to a continuous slow pattern. By 41 weeks, occipital lambda waves are sometimes present with visual fixation.

EEG FROM FULL TERM TO ADOLESCENCE

In order to understand the EEG in children we emphasize that variability is the rule – certainly much greater than in adults. The late neonatal features discussed earlier, multifocal sharp waves, tracé alternant, and frontal sharp waves, are rarely seen past 44 weeks CA.

During the first year of life there is a gradual shift from delta to theta. Over the next 2 years, delta declines markedly, and at about 3 years there is predominately diffuse theta with less frequent delta waves. Between ages 3 and 6 years, diffuse theta declines further. By age 8 years some theta persists, as it does for the next few years. This is where confusion arises. We find a wide range of theta prominence in young subjects with no demonstrable cerebral pathology on imaging studies and no neurological deficits. Thus, unless there is some clinical correlation for "excessive" slowing, particularly in the theta range, it is best to be generous. When in doubt, opt for a declaration of normal rather than abnormal. On the other hand, if there is a great deal of delta after age 4 or 5 years, the odds are that there indeed is cerebral dysfunction. Observe that diffuse slowing, regardless of degree, must be symmetric. Asymmetric slowing is indicative of cerebral dysfunction. Note: It is particularly important to obtain a true waking record in children. They are frequently drowsy or rapidly become so. Thus, assessment of slowing must be made during the alert state.

AWAKE EEG

The posterior dominant rhythm (PDR) is not present at birth but begins in the majority of infants to appear in the third or fourth month of life and is 3–4 Hz (Figure 3-6). This rhythm, like its adult counterpart, is present in the wakeful state when the eyes are closed and attenuates with eye opening. At 6 months, for most infants, the PDR is 5 Hz; at 12 months, the PDR is 6 Hz; and at 36 months, the majority of children will have a PDR of 8 Hz (Figure 3-7). (Hint: It is easier to remember if you start with a PDR of 8 Hz at the age of 3 years and then work backwards – 8 Hz: 3 years, 7 Hz: 2 years, 6 Hz: 1 year, 5 Hz: 6 months, 3–4 Hz: 3–4 months). Between 3 years of age and adulthood, the PDR shifts higher in the alpha range (8–13 Hz) and should exceed 8.5 Hz in adults. The amplitude of the PDR is often asymmetric, typically higher in amplitude on the right (the skull on the left is often thicker, conveniently protecting our left dominant brain). This is normal, as long as the higher amplitude is not greater than two times the lower amplitude.

FEATURES OF SLEEP

In the term infant, the background pattern of quiet sleep transitions from a tracé alternant pattern to a pattern of continuous high-voltage slow activity. In a normal infant, sleep architecture typically begins to develop at 1.5–3 months with the appearance of sleep spindles. These early sleep spindles are several seconds in duration, in a frontocentral location, in the high alpha or low beta range, and are not synchronous (Figure 3-8). The lack of synchrony is likely due to lack of myelination in the neonatal brain. By 2 years of age, it is considered abnormal if most spindles are still asynchronous (Figure 3-9). Persistent absence of sleep spindles on one side raises the suspicious for ipsilateral dysfunction. Sleep spindles are part of stage II sleep.

Vertex waves and K-complexes should be well developed by 5–6 months. They can have a similar distribution, both maximal at the vertex of the head. The vertex waves phase reverses, often at the C3 or C4 electrodes in a bipolar montage, and can occur in repetitive runs, particularly in children (Figure 3-10). Vertex waves have a shorter duration, <200 ms, while K-complexes are often >500 ms. Vertex waves can be seen in stage I and II sleep and K-complexes (like sleep spindles) are part of stage II sleep. K-complexes occur spontaneously and in response to stimulation, particularly noise.

By 3 months of age, infants typically have a sleep onset consisting of non-REM sleep, which is typical of the normal adult. In addition, REM sleep begins to occupy a lower percentage of total sleep time, going from 50% at full term to 40% at 3 months and finally 20% in the adolescent and adult. Within the first year of life the EEG begins to show sleep stages similar to those of the adult with REM, stage I, stage II, and slow wave sleep (SWS).

NORMAL VARIANTS

Half alpha variant

In wake, there are a few normal variants typically not seen in adults. The half alpha variant can be seen in children typically after the age of 8. As the name suggests, it is approximately one half the frequency of the PDR and often has a notched appearance (Figure 3-11).

Posterior slow waves of youth

Posterior slow waves of youth occur commonly between 2 and 21 years of age (Figure 3-12). They are typically in the delta range, consisting of 3–6 fused alpha waves. Both half alpha variant and posterior slow waves of youth should attenuate with eye opening and alerting stimulation.

Hypnogogic/hypnopompic hypersynchrony

In drowsiness, between the ages of 6 months and 2 years, most children will develop a pattern with bursts of diffuse, high voltage (>350 μV),

Text continued on p. 84

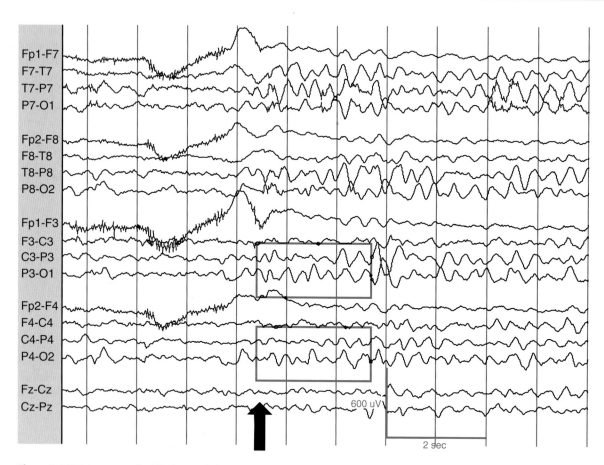

Figure 3-6 PDR in a 4-month-old infant. Well-formed PDR (boxes) of 3–4 Hz, which is brought out by eye closure (arrow).

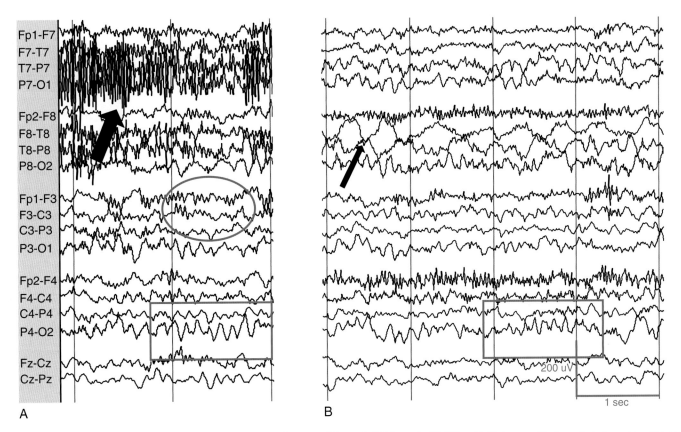

A   B

Figure 3-7 PDR in two 2-year-old children. Both (**A**) and (**B**) show a well-formed PDR (boxes) of 7–8 Hz with higher amplitude posteriorly and lower amplitude anteriorly. In (**A**), there is abundant jaw artifact (thick arrow) and low amplitude beta activity is superimposed on theta anteriorly (oval). (**B**) There is pacifier artifact seen at T8 (thin arrow).

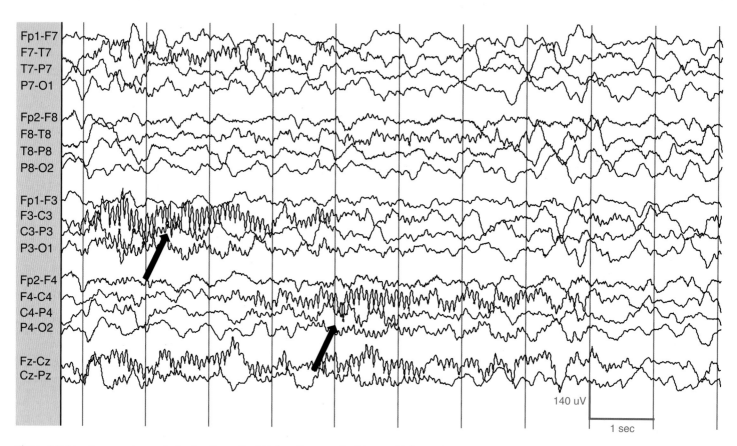

Figure 3-8 Asynchronous sleep spindles in a 2-month-old infant. Two-month-old normal infant with well-formed asynchronous sleep spindles (arrows). Rule of 2: at 2 months of age sleep spindles appear but are asynchronous. At 2 years of age sleep spindles become synchronous.

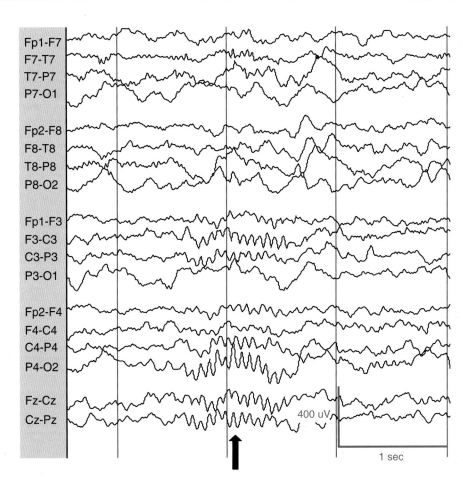

Figure 3-9 Synchronous sleep spindles in an 18-month-old infant.

400 uV

1 sec

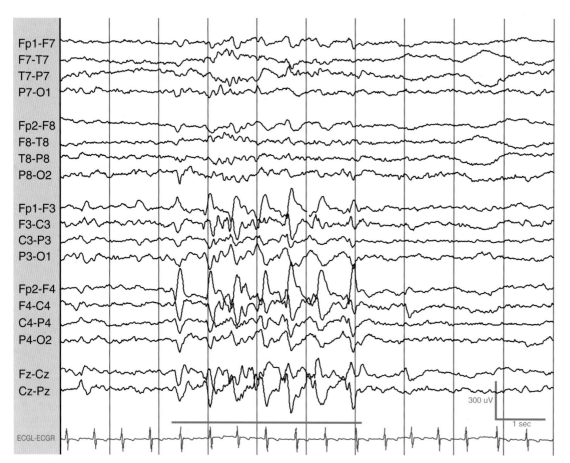

Figure 3-10 Vertex waves. 3-year-old girl with a repetitive run of vertex waves (line).

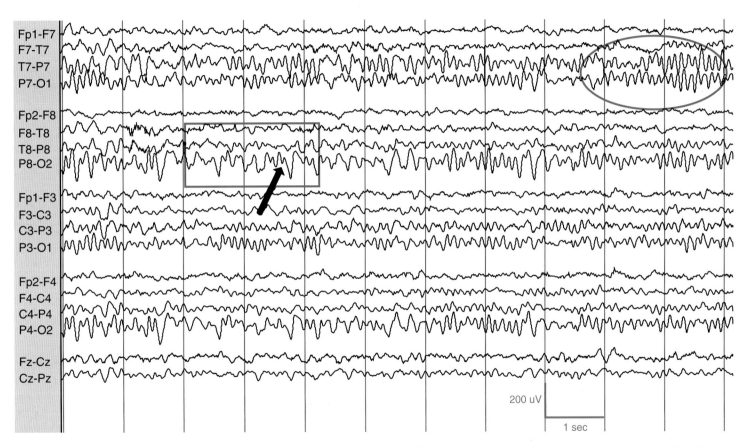

Figure 3-11 Half alpha variant. 8-year-old girl with a normal PDR of 8 Hz (oval). A typical half alpha variant of 4 Hz is present (rectangle), more on the right, with a characteristic notched morphology (arrow).

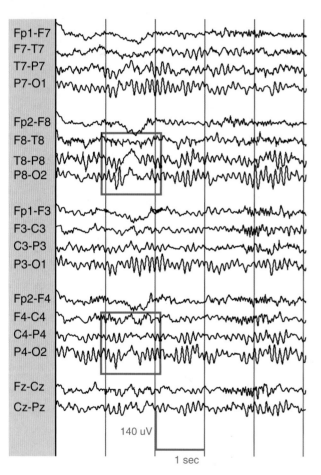

Figure 3-12 Posterior slow waves of youth. 7-year-old boy with a well-formed PDR of 9 Hz with a posterior slow wave of youth seen on the right (boxes).

slow waves (3–5 Hz) lasting for several seconds: Hypnogogic hypersynchrony. An identical pattern, termed hypnopompic hypersynchrony (Figure 3-13), can be seen with transitions from sleep to wake. These patterns are not often seen after adolescence. By approximately age 10, children can have slow roving lateral eye movements in drowsiness. This persists throughout adulthood.

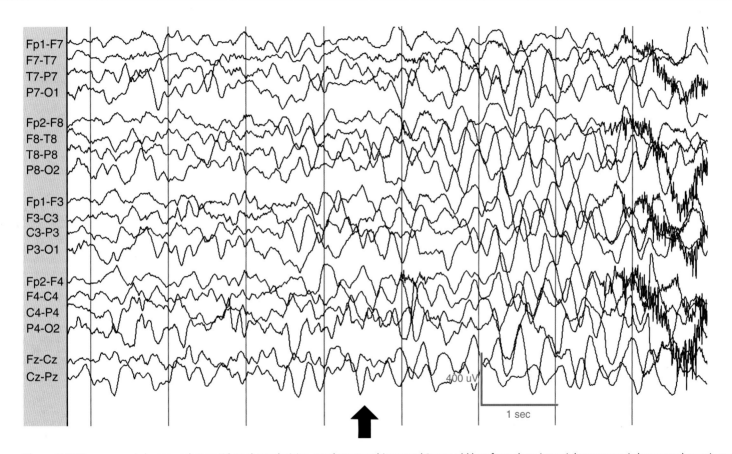

Figure 3-13 Hypnopompic hypersynchrony. When the technician gently rouses this normal 2-year-old boy from sleep (arrow), hypnopompic hypersynchrony is seen with high voltage 3 Hz activity.

Further reading

Battin, M., Rutherford, M., 2001. Magnetic resonance imaging of the brain in preterm infants: 24 weeks' gestation to term. In: Rutherford, M.A. (Ed.), MRI of the Neonatal Brain. WB Saunders, London. (Part 2, Chapter 3).

Blum, W.T., 1982. Atlas of Pediatric EEG. Raven, New York.

Eeg-Olofsson, O., 1971. The development of the electroencephalogram in normal adolescents from the age of 16 through 21 years. Neuropädiatrie 3, 11–45.

Fisch, B.J., 1999. The normal EEG from premature age to the age of 19 years. In: Fisch, B.J. (Ed.), Fisch and Spehlmann's EEG Primer. Elsevier, Oxford, pp. 155–184.

Laoprasert, P., 2011. Atlas of Pediatric EEG. McGraw Hill, London, pp. 201–273.

Marcuse, L.V., Schneider, M., Mortati, K.A., et al., 2008. Quantitative analysis of the EEG posterior-dominant rhythm in healthy adolescents. Clin. Neurophysiol. 119 (8), 1778–1781. doi:10.1016/j.clinph.2008.02.023.

Petersen, I., Eeg-Olofsson, O., 1971. The development of the electroencephalogram in normal children from the age of 1 through 15 years. Nonparoxysmal activity. Neuropädiatrie 2, 247–304.

Tharp, B.R., 1980. Neonatal and pediatric electroencephalography. In: Aminoff, M.J. (Ed.), Electrodiagnosis in Clinical Neurology. Churchill-Livingstone, New York, pp. 67–117.

Tsuchida, T.N., Wusthoff, C.J., Shelhass, R.A., et al. American Clinical Neurophysiology Society standardized EEG terminology and categorization for the description of continuous EEG monitoring in neonates: report of the American Clinical Neurophysiology Society Critical Care Monitoring Committee.

Westmoreland, B.F., Klass, D.W., 1996. Electroencephalography: Electroencephalograms of neonates, infants and children. In: Daube, J. (Ed.), Clinical Neurophysiology. FA Davis, Philadelphia, pp. 104–113.

BACKGROUND ABNORMALITIES

ORGANIZATION

In the awake state, in a well-organized EEG, there is a well-formed posterior dominant rhythm (PDR) occipitally, which attenuates with eye opening. Anteriorly, the frequencies are faster and lower in amplitude. This is sometimes referred to as the normal anterior-posterior (A-P) gradient. In sleep, there are distinct sleep states with sleep structures (e.g., K-complexes, vertex waves) specific to each state. If these elements are entirely lacking, the EEG is said to be poorly organized. If an individual has some elements of normal organization but not all, the organization is described as fair.

DIFFUSE SLOWING

The presence of diffuse slowing suggests bilateral cerebral dysfunction with a broad spectrum of causes. The first major problem in making a determination of diffuse slowing is the patient's state of alertness. Many patients are quite drowsy throughout a routine EEG recording. This, of course, produces slowing of the record that would not necessarily be abnormal. The electroencephalographer must diagnose the presence of diffuse slowing during the most alert segments of recording. If this is not possible, one may have to say that the diffuse slowing may be in part, if not wholly, due to drowsiness, although a degree of cerebral pathology cannot be excluded. For patients with a depressed level of consciousness, the degree of slowing is determined after an alerting stimuli (often nailbed pressure) (Figure 4-1).

When an alert segment is encountered, the PDR, if present, is determined. In adults, a PDR of 8.5 Hz or less is abnormal. If the abnormal PDR is symmetric, this is usually not secondary to a focal (i.e., posterior) problem, but a diffuse abnormality. In addition, abundant theta in the awake adult record or abundant delta in the awake child record usually indicates diffuse slowing, which correlates with either diffuse or multifocal cerebral dysfunction.

In adults, mild slowing is used if the primary background frequency is in the high theta range (7–8 Hz), moderate slowing is used if the frequencies are mainly in the mid theta range (4–7 Hz), and severe slowing is used if the frequencies are mainly in the delta range (0–<4 Hz). Of note, diffuse slowing does not always correlate with the degree of cerebral dysfunction. The classic example of this is in alpha coma where there is no slowing but there is severe cerebral dysfunction.

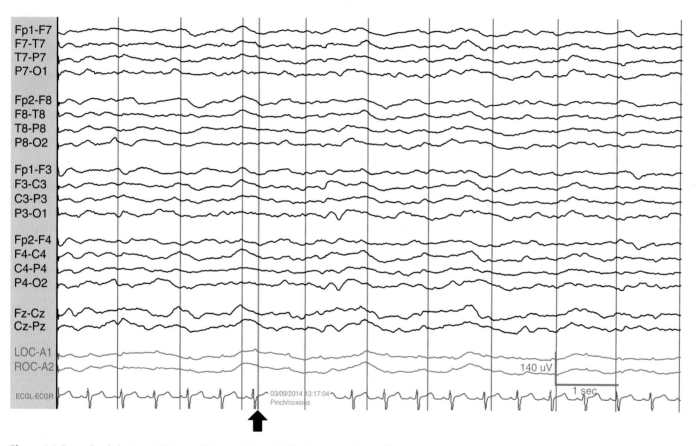

Figure 4-1 Generalized slowing. A 46-year-old man with sepsis. The background is poorly organized without a PDR. There is generalized background slowing, consisting mainly of delta frequencies. There is no EEG reactivity to noxious stimulus (arrow).

A second problem relates to medication. We encounter this frequently, especially with referrals from psychiatry. Many psychotropic drugs (e.g., phenothiazines, lithium and clozapine) can cause diffuse slowing. While it is true that the record is abnormal in such cases, the patient may demonstrate no obvious neurological dysfunction. Thus, when reporting this abnormality, it is important to state that the background slowing may be due to an effect of medication(s) that the patient is taking.

Many pathologic processes lead to diffuse slowing, as well as slowing of the PDR. Alzheimer's disease, multi-infarct dementia, various toxic-metabolic disorders, post-ictal states, and congenital brain damage come to mind.

FOCAL SLOWING

As we have seen, slow waves in and of themselves are not abnormal, but slowing that is localized or lateralized commands our attention. In fact, the EEG is highly sensitive to the presence of localized cerebral pathology, often more so than imaging studies. The most important focal abnormality is delta activity (0–<4 Hz) occurring in any cerebral location. Focal delta waves are a good indicator of structural disease. At times focal delta may not correlate with an evident structural lesion on MRI/CT studies, even though cerebral pathology of some degree underlies the EEG finding (e.g., frontotemporal slowing in non-lesional temporal lobe epilepsy).

Structural lesions producing focal delta include brain tumors, cerebral infarction, brain abscess, subdural hematoma, intracerebral hemorrhage, and other traumatic brain injuries. Focal rhythmic (monomorphic) and polymorphic delta activity can be present interictally in patients with focal seizures, with or without clear structural lesions. Delta foci are often most evident in the temporal derivations, even when the main pathology is not in the temporal lobe. We term this false localization, the slowing being projected to the temporal regions from deeper or adjacent structures.

When examining focal slowing, the prevalence of the abnormality should be noted according to ACNS guidelines (Table 4-1). For example, if the slowing is present for 10–49% percent of the EEG, it is described as frequent.

Polymorphic delta is thought to be generated from lesions involving the white matter (Figure 4-2). Contrast this with rhythmic delta activity that can result from lesions of gray matter – usually cortical. Polymorphic and rhythmic delta often coexist when lesions involve both cortex and subcortical white matter.

FOCAL ATTENUATION

Fast activity is believed to be generated at the level of cerebral cortex, so focal attenuation of fast activity is a useful marker of abnormal cortical function. It can happen in acute cortical injury such as ischemic stroke. It can also occur in the setting of an intervening fluid collection between the scalp and the brain, such as a subdural hematoma (Figure 4-3).

Focal increased fast activity

Focal increased fast activity can be present in the setting of brain abscess, stroke, tumors, vascular malformations, and cortical dysplasia. Interestingly, these can all be associated with focal decrease in fast activity as well. It needs to be differentiated from the breach artifact, which results from an area of skull defect, usually a postsurgical finding. In the case of a breach artifact, the waveforms are often sharply contoured at higher amplitudes. The technicians are asked to note the presence of craniotomy scars in order to correctly identify this rhythm. Due to the prior surgery, breach rhythms are often associated with focal slowing (Figure 4-4).

Text continued on p. 96

Table 4-1 ACNS Standardized Critical Care EEG Terminology

Main term 1	Main term 2	Plus (+) modifier
G *Generalized* • Optional: specify frontally, midline or occipitally predominant	**PD** *Periodic discharges*	**No +**
	RDA *Rhythmic delta activity*	**F+** *Superimposed fast activity–applies to PD or RDA only*
L *Lateralized* • Optional: specify unilateral or bilateral asymmetric • Optional: specify lobe(s) most involved or hemispheric	**SW** *Rhythmic spike and wave* *or* *rhythmic sharp and slow wave* *or* *rhythmic polyspike and wave*	**+R** *Superimposed rhythmic activity–applies to PD only*
		+S *Superimposed sharp waves or spikes, or sharply contoured–applies to RDA only*
BI *Bilateral independent* • Optional: specify symmetric or asymmetric • Optional: specify lobe(s) most involved or hemispheric		**+FR** *If both subtypes apply–applies to PD only*
		+FS *If both subtypes apply–applies to RDA only*
Mf *Multifocal* • Optional: specify symmetric or asymmetric • Optional: specify lobe(s) most involved or hemispheric		

Continued

Table 4-1 continued

Major modifiers

Prevalence	Duration	Frequency	Phases[1]	Sharpness[2]	Absolute amplitude	Relative amplitude[3]	Polarity[2]	Stimulus induced	Evolution[4]
Continuous ≥90%	Very long ≥1 h	≥4/s	>3	Spiky <70 ms	High ≥200 µV	>2	Negative	**SI** *stimulus induced*	Evolving
Abundant 50-89%	Long 5–59 min	3.5/s	3	Sharp 70-200 ms	Medium 50–199 µV	≤2	Positive	**Sp** *Spontaneous only*	Fluctuating
Frequent 10-49%	Intermediate duration 1–4.9 min	3/s	2	Sharply contoured >200 ms	Low 20–49 µV		Dipole	**Unk** *Unknown*	Static
Occasional 1-9%	Brief 10-59 s	2.5/s	1	Blunt >200 ms	Very low <20 µV		Unclear		
Rare <1%	Very brief <10 s	2/s							
		1.5/s							
		1/s							
		0.5/s							
		<0.5/s							

Minor modifiers

Onset	Triphasic[5]	Lag
Sudden ≤3 s	Yes	**A-P** *Anterior-posterior*
Gradual >3 s	No	**P-A** *Posterior-anterior*
		No

NOTE 1: Applies to PD and SW only, including the slow wave of the SW complex
NOTE 2: Applies to the predominant phase of PD and the spike or sharp component of SW only
NOTE 3: Applies to PD only
NOTE 4: Refers to frequency, location or morphology
NOTE 5: Applies to PD or SW only

Continued

Table 4-1 continued

Sporadic epileptiform discharges	Background									
Prevalence	Symmetry	Breach effect	PDR	Background EEG frequency	AP gradient	Variability	Reactivity	Voltage	Stage II sleep transients	Continuity
Abundant ≥1/10 s										
Frequent 1/min–1/10 s	Symmetric	Present	Present Specify frequency	Delta	Present	Present	Present	Normal ≥20 µV	Present and normal	Continuous
Occasional 1/h–1/min										
Rare <1/h	Mild asymmetry ≤50% amp. 0.5–1/s freq.	Absent	Absent	Theta	Absent	Absent	SIRPIDs only	Low 10–20 µV	Present but abnormal	Nearly continuous: ≤10% periods of suppression (<10 µV) or attenuation (≥10 µV but <50% of background voltage)
	Marked asymmetry >50% amp. >1/s freq.	Unclear		≥Alpha	Reverse	Unclear	Absent	Suppressed <10 µV	Absent	Discontinuous: 10–49% periods of suppression or attenuation
							Unclear			Burst-suppression or Burst-attenuation: 50–99% periods of suppression or attenuation
										Suppression

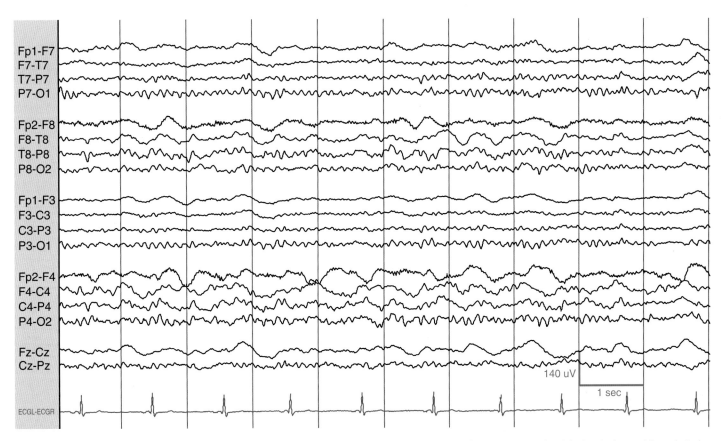

Figure 4-2 Focal slowing. A 27-year-old woman with a right-sided brain tumor. Note polymorphic delta frequencies over the right hemisphere, with a relatively preserved posterior dominant rhythm.

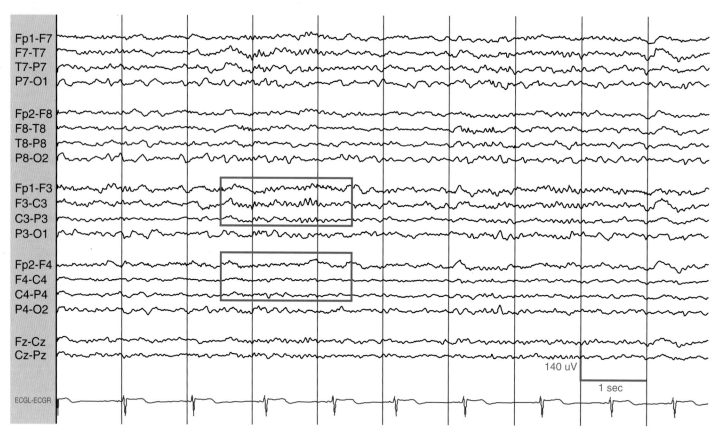

Figure 4-3 Focal attenuation. A 66-year-old woman who presented with an acute right-sided subdural hematoma. There is attenuation of fast frequencies over the right side, compared with the left side (boxes).

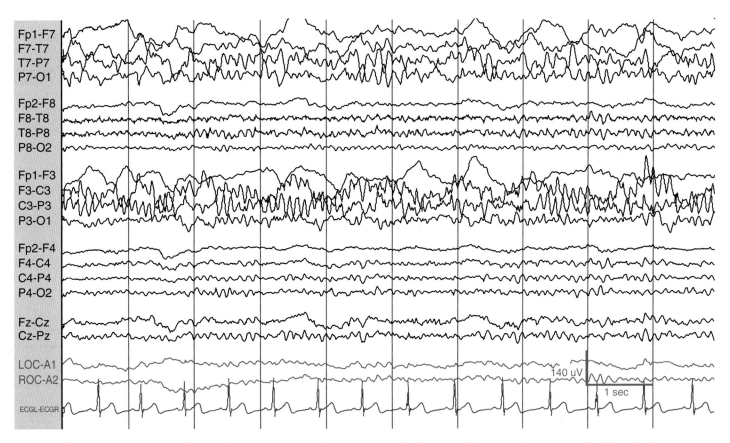

Figure 4-4 Breach rhythm. A 21-year-old man with a history of traumatic brain injury and brain surgery. There is focal slowing over the left hemisphere, and a breach rhythm is seen most prominently over the left frontoparietal region.

95

EPILEPTIFORM DISCHARGES, PERIODIC OR RHYHMIC PATTERNS

EPILEPTIFORM DISCHARGES

In patients with epilepsy, despite the important role of the EEG, the diagnosis often rests on clinical grounds. Rarely, epileptiform discharges can be recorded in persons without epilepsy. Likewise, patients with epilepsy can have a normal EEG between seizures. Nonetheless, the EEG provides important supporting evidence for a diagnosis of epilepsy. Moreover, the type of epilepsy may be confirmed, or even diagnosed. For example, the EEG differentiates between focal and generalized epilepsies and is a principal feature in the definition of epilepsy syndromes.

The following paragraphs provide direction concerning specific findings in epilepsy.

The spike, the spike-wave complex and polyspikes

The spike is defined as a paroxysmal potential (i.e., it arises suddenly from the background) that is very sharp in contour (you can prick your finger on it) and whose rise has a steeper slope than that of its decline. Its duration is 20 to 70 ms, thus differentiating it from more rapid muscle action potentials. Spikes are usually electronegative at the surface, although there are exceptions. The spike is usually followed by a low-voltage slow potential (duration of about 200 ms) before the baseline is re-established. In some cases the slow wave may not be evident. Spikes may occur in isolation, in groups of two or more, or in repetitive runs (Figure 4-5). They may be focal, multifocal or generalized.

The spike-wave complex consists of two components – the spike and the accompanying time-locked slow wave. The prototype is the generalized spike-wave complex recorded in patients with absence epilepsy (Figure 4-6). In this case the complex is in the 3 Hz frequency band. The discharge is relatively high in voltage (say 200–300 μV or more), and the slow wave is usually higher in amplitude than the spike. Both the spike and wave are surface negative. A polyspike-wave is a series of spikes occurring before the slow wave (Figure 4-7). Another distinctive pattern is the generalized irregular polyspike-wave discharge at 4–6 Hz, characteristic of juvenile myoclonic epilepsy (JME).

Spike-wave complexes also occur at frequencies other than 3 Hz. The prototype of slow spike-wave (1.5–2.5 Hz) occurs in Lennox–Gastaut syndrome (LGS) and is generalized at times with a bifrontal preponderance.

The sharp wave

The sharp wave is defined as a paroxysmal sharp potential (not as pointed as a spike) that has a duration of 70 to 200 ms (Figure 4-8). The duration cutoff between spikes and sharp waves is somewhat arbitrary, and the clinical significance is not so different; however, certain epilepsy syndromes have characteristic epileptiform potentials. A sharp wave is typically followed by a slow wave.

Other interictal paroxysmal waveforms

Patients with long-standing epilepsy and generalized seizures, possibly in remission, commonly have generalized irregular slow-wave discharges, sometimes with sharp components. Patients with absence epilepsy may demonstrate brief rhythmic high-voltage 3 Hz slow-wave discharges without accompanying spikes. Such discharges probably represent a forme fruste of 3 Hz spike-wave activity.

Brief potentially ictal rhythmic discharges (BIRDs) are very brief (<10 seconds) runs of focal or generalized rhythmic activity greater than 4 Hz without evolution. They typically last for 0.5–4 seconds (Figure 4-9).

Text continued on p. 102

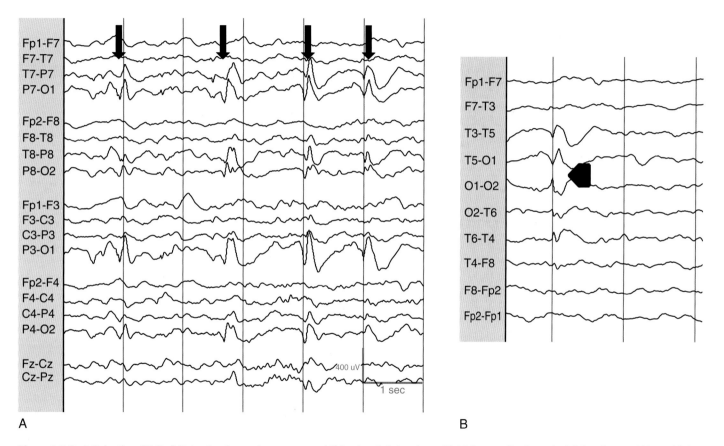

A

B

Figure 4-5 Occipital spikes. (**A**) Occipital spikes (arrows) are seen over bilateral occipital regions with higher amplitude on the left in a 6-year-old boy with late-onset childhood occipital epilepsy. (**B**) In the circumferential montage, a phase reversal at O1 is seen (arrowhead).

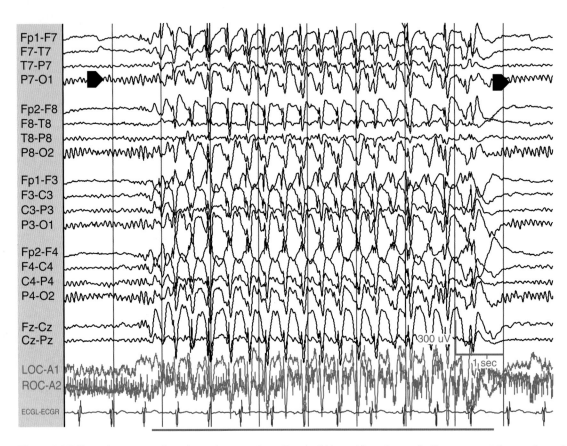

Figure 4-6 Spike and wave complexes in an absence seizure. 7-year-old boy with staring spells. You can count three spike and wave complexes per second (3 Hz spike and wave) (line). Before and after the spike wave complexes a clear PDR of 11 Hz can be appreciated (arrowhead).

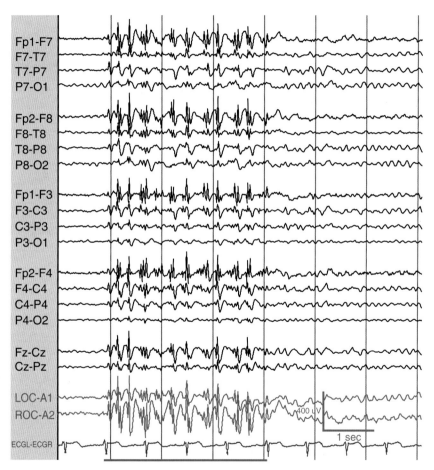

Figure 4-7 Polyspike and wave. 9-year-old girl with GTCC with 3 Hz generalized polyspike and wave for 3 seconds (line).

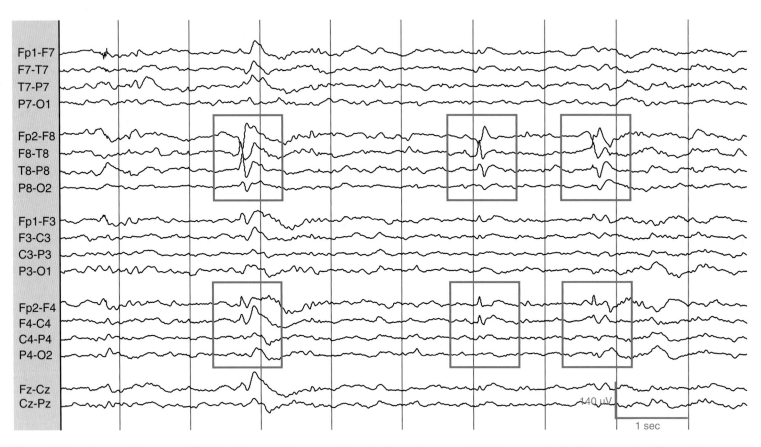

Figure 4-8 Frontotemporal sharp waves. Right frontotemporal sharp waves (boxes), with maximum negativity (phase reversing) at F8, are seen in a 33-year-old woman with right mesial temporal sclerosis.

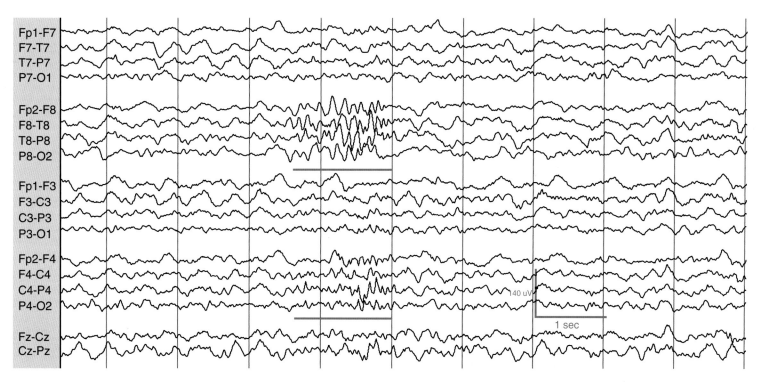

Figure 4-9 Brief potential ictal rhythmic discharges (BIRDs). Rhythmic 1.5-second right hemispheric theta and alpha activity (line) in a 25-year-old man with focal epilepsy of right hemisphere origin.

They are associated with high risk of seizures and are highly correlated with the seizure focus. These discharges can display rapid bisynchrony and appear generalized even when a focal source is known.

Generalized paroxysmal fast activity (GPFA), which could be considered as a type of BIRDs, consists of diffuse >12 Hz activity often with a frontal predominance lasting typically between 2 and 10 seconds (Figure 4-10). These bursts can be interictal, but close correlation with clinical behavior is warranted as tonic seizures can be very subtle clinically. GPFA is commonly seen in patients with LGS during sleep.

LOCATION AND SIGNIFICANCE OF FOCAL EPILEPTIFORM DISCHARGES

Temporal epileptiform discharges

The most common sites for focal epileptiform activity are the temporal lobes. In patients with temporal lobe epilepsy the discharges may be maximal in the anterior temporal regions (F7/F8 electrodes) (Figure 4-8). Of note, the F7/F8 electrodes also record spikes originating from the inferior frontal cortex. Note, however, that temporal lobe discharges may demonstrate a focal maximum between the anterior and mid-temporal electrodes (F7/T7 or F8/T8), or indeed at the mid-temporal electrodes (T7/T8). Some laboratories employ F9 and F10 electrodes, placed inferior to F7/F8. The temporal lobe spike may be more evident and of higher amplitude at these locations.

The majority of patients with temporal lobe epilepsy will have interictal epileptiform discharges. The frequency of recorded discharges, however, has a weak correlation with the patient's seizure control, although it is true that the number of discharges tends to decline in persistently seizure-free patients.

If epileptiform discharges are present bilaterally in the temporal lobes, it is difficult to determine, on grounds of the EEG, which temporal lobe generates the clinical seizure activity. The more active focus may not be responsible for the patient's recurrent seizures as has been shown with intensive video-EEG monitoring. Alternatively, the seizures may emanate from either temporal lobe at various times.

Mid-temporal epileptiform discharges may have a different significance than discharges that are more anterior. Such discharges are seen after significant head trauma or with a temporal lobe tumor, resulting in damage to the temporal cortex.

Note that posterior temporal/parietal epileptiform discharges (P7/P8) usually result from more posterior temporal cortical damage and may result from infarction or other pathology in the region of the posterior cerebral circulation.

Occipital epileptiform discharges

The occipital epileptiform discharge focus (O1/O2) is distinctive and usually found in children with occipital epilepsy (see Table 5-2, epilepsy syndromes). Care must be taken in discovering its existence for it is easy to concentrate on other brain areas, particularly the temporal regions, and neglect the occipital regions save for determining the frequency of the PDR. This is especially true when the spikes are infrequent, for they are easily obscured by ongoing background activity. Important to note is the downward deviation of the epileptiform discharges in the occipital channels in the longitudinal bipolar montage. There is no phase-reversal because the occipital electrode is the last in the chain.

An electrode arrangement (montage) that is useful in recording occipital events is referred to as the circumferential montage. Here, the electrodes are linked around the scalp, running through the occipital and frontopolar regions. Thus, any occipital spike will demonstrate a phase reversal at O1 or O2 (Figure 4-5). A referential montage can be useful as well and will simply demonstrate the highest amplitude at the occipital electrode. Note also that occipital epileptiform discharges may manifest in

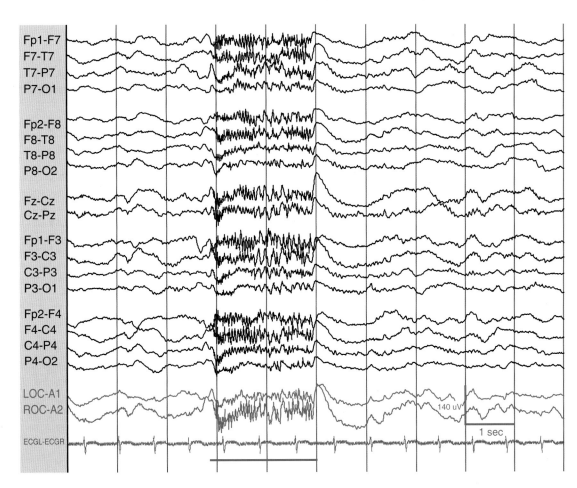

Figure 4-10 Generalized paroxysmal fast activity (GPFA). GPFA (line) in a 21-year-old woman with focal epilepsy (seizures with right head turn with right arm extension). All of her epileptiform discharges appear generalized (like this one), likely representing rapid bisynchrony. There was no clinical correlate during this particular discharge.

both occipital regions, the side of higher amplitude being the putative focus.

The clinical history may help in directing attention to the occipital regions inasmuch as such patients may report visual symptoms consisting of bright or flashing lights or a grid pattern (not formed visual hallucinations such as scenes or persons). Formed visual hallucinations (e.g., "I see my grandmother wearing that floral apron") occur in patients with focal seizures of temporal neocortical origin. The EEG diagnosis is important in that occipital epilepsy presenting in childhood usually has a favorable prognosis, both for immediate seizure control and eventual seizure subsidence. The same may not apply to adults.

Centrotemporal epileptiform discharges

Centrotemporal epileptiform discharges are distinctive and, once seen, are not forgotten. They are the accompaniment of benign epilepsy of childhood with centrotemporal spikes (BECTS). The discharges are clearly focal, with a maximum negativity (i.e., phase reversal) at the centrotemporal area (C3/T7, C4/T8). Alternatively, the discharges may be maximal in the central and parietal areas (C3/P3, C4/P4), and occipital spikes may co-exist. Characteristically, there is a horizontal dipole: negative maxima in the centrotemporal electrodes and positive maxima in the frontal area (Figure 4-11). They are best seen in the average referential montage. It means that the spike generator is located tangential to the surface electrode as opposed to perpendicular (like most other spike discharges).

Frontal and frontopolar epileptiform discharges

These discharges can be recorded in patients with seizures originating in either frontal lobe or with generalized seizures. The frontopolar epileptiform discharge (Fp1/Fp2) is thought to be generated by orbital frontal cortex or adjacent areas, whereas the frontal epileptiform discharge at the mid-frontal electrode(s) (F3/F4) is generated by the frontal convexity. For example, a right frontopolar spike when recorded on a longitudinal bipolar montage is an up-going potential in channels Fp2/F8 and Fp2/F4. As in the case of occipital spikes, there is no phase reversal (Fp1/2 are the first electrodes in the chain). These discharges are well displayed with the circumferential montage (Figure 4-12). As with occipital spikes, there is often representation in the opposite hemisphere at lower voltage. In addition, a focal frontal epilepsy may have interictal discharges that are bilaterally synchronous with equal amplitude on both sides. In addition, an individual with generalized epilepsy may have spike fragments that are lateralized and frontally predominant. To make matters more confusing, a right mesial frontal focus may create a spike on the EEG that phase reverses on the left, say at the F3 electrode. This is because the synchronous excitatory post synaptic potentials (EPSPs) responsible for any epileptiform discharge create a negative charge along the cortical surface. When that cortical surface is in the mesial right frontal lobe, the negative dipole may project best onto the left frontocentral area, simply because of geometry. When this occurs it is called false lateralization.

Midline epileptiform discharges

We often say that, during drowsiness or sleep, any sharp potential discharge occurring at one of the midline electrodes should be regarded as a normal phenomenon (vertex sharp waves) unless proven otherwise. However, epilepsy foci on the mesial surface of the cerebral hemispheres can cause interictal discharges which are maximal at midline electrodes (Fz, Cz, or Pz). Distinguishing between an epileptiform abnormality and a vertex wave can be difficult. If midline spikes are seen in wakefulness, they are definitely abnormal.

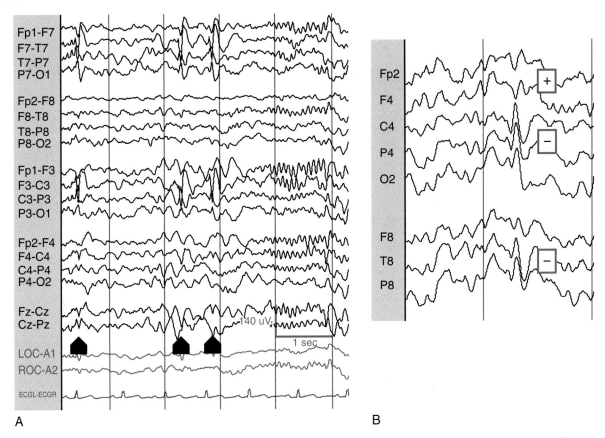

Figure 4-11 Benign epilepsy with centrotemporal spikes (BECTS). (**A**) Left centrotemporal spikes in repetitive runs are seen in sleep (note spindles) in an 8-year-old boy with BECTS. (**B**) A right-sided centrotemporal spike in an average montage. Fp2 and F4 are electropositive (downward deflection) and C4, P4, and T8 are electronegative (upward deflection) on the average montage. This is the horizontal dipole.

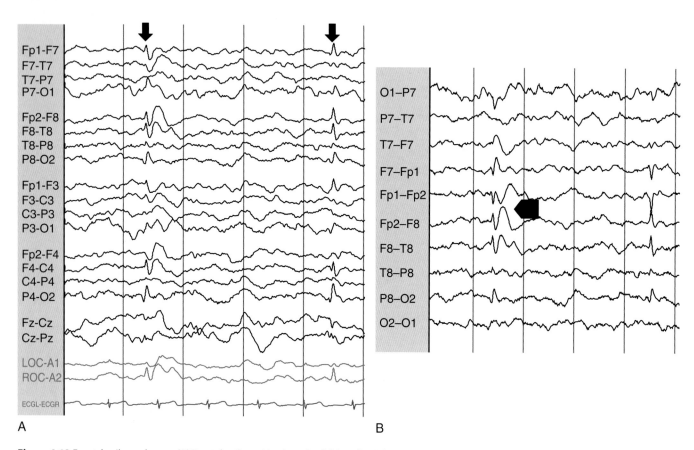

A

B

Figure 4-12 Frontal spike and wave. (**A**) Frontal spikes with a broader field on the right are seen in a 5-year-old girl. (**B**) On the circumferential montage (right side), phase reversal at Fp2 is seen.

RHYTHMIC PATTERNS

These patterns can be seen in patients with epilepsy, but they are more commonly seen in patients who are critically ill. Nowadays, continuous EEG monitoring is more commonly and widely used to assess brain function in critically ill patients, and these patterns are frequently encountered. In order to facilitate communication and aid in further research, the American Clinical Neurophysiology Society has published and revised the standardized ICU EEG nomenclature, which is used in the following discussions (Table 4-1, p. 89). Here we will focus on generalized and lateralized rhythmic and periodic patterns.

Generalized rhythmic delta activity (GRDA)

The term GRDA is used to describe repetitive waveforms that are generalized, monomorphic, and rhythmic in the delta frequency (Figure 4-13). Frontally predominant GRDA (aka, FIRDA; frontal intermittent rhythmic delta activity) is most typically seen in adults, whereas occipitally predominant GRDA (aka, OIRDA; occipital intermittent rhythmic delta activity) is more commonly seen in children. The occipitally predominant GRDA is often seen in children with absence epilepsy. Frontally predominant GRDA is a more non-specific pattern and can be indicative of a toxic-metabolic encephalopathy, a process that involves deep midline structures, subcortical or cortical structural lesions, and/or raised intracranial pressure. It must be differentiated from repetitive eye blink artifact (Figure 1-18). A differential point is posterior extension of the potential field in the case of frontally predominant GRDA while eye blink artifact is usually confined to the frontal regions. Most laboratories employ two periorbital electrodes, one on the lateral lower aspect of the left canthus and the other on the lateral upper aspect of the right canthus. During eye blinks, these eye leads will be mirror images of each other while during frontally predominant GRDA the eye leads will be synchronous and symmetric.

Lateralized rhythmic delta activity (LRDA)

When the RDA lateralizes to one side of the brain, it is termed LRDA. LRDA can be present in any particular lobe (frontal, parietal, temporal, occipital) or may appear broadly in one hemisphere (Figure 4-14). According to ACNS critical care EEG terminology, if there is bilateral synchronous RDA with a clear predominance of one hemisphere, it is termed LRDA, bilateral asymmetric. LRDA is most often seen when there is a lesion in the gray matter and is often associated with focal cerebral hyperexcitability.

PERIODIC PATTERNS

This EEG term refers to a periodic pattern consisting of discharges occurring at more or less fixed intervals. Periodic discharges are indicative of significant cerebral disease, whether focal or generalized.

GENERALIZED PERIODIC DISCHARGES (GPDs)

These are generalized, synchronous discharges that recur at a certain interval. The discharges vary in waveform but are usually characterized by synchronous high-voltage spikes or sharp waves. GPDs (aka GPEDs; generalized periodic epileptiform discharges) are usually accompanied by a severely abnormal background because of some underlying process that is causing severe bihemispheric dysfunction (Figure 4-15). In general, GPDs can be seen in a diverse array of clinical conditions including hypoxic-ischemic encephalopathy, severe toxic-metabolic encephalopathy, Creutzfeldt–Jakob disease (CJD), or subacute sclerosing panencephalitis (SSPE), which is caused by the measles virus (rare now thanks to vaccination). GPDs, particularly in a toxic metabolic encephalopathy, may have a triphasic morphology and can have an anterior to posterior

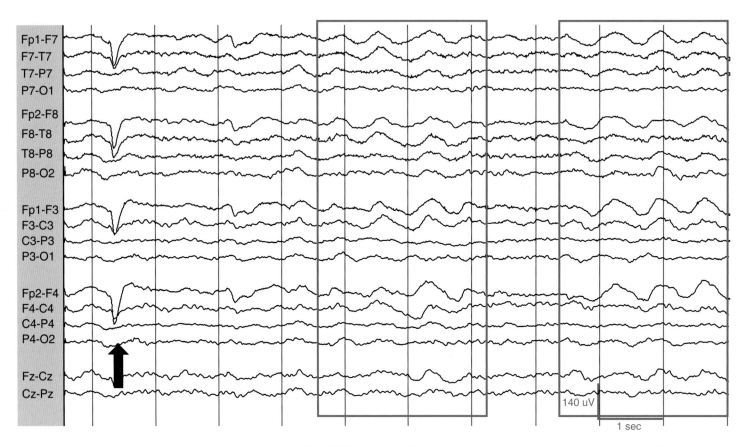

Figure 4-13 Frontally predominant generalized rhythmic delta activity (GRDA). A 32-year-old man who developed fever and altered mental status after a small bowel resection. After an eye blink artifact (arrow), frontally predominant GRDA at 1 Hz is shown (boxes).

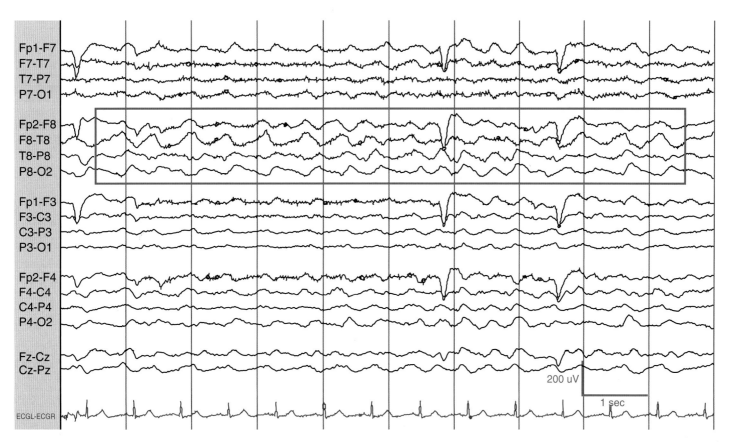

Figure 4-14 Lateralized rhythmic delta activity (LRDA). A 63-year-old man with a history of multifocal strokes presented with acute altered mental status. Rhythmic delta activity is seen over the right hemisphere, most prominently over the temporal chain.

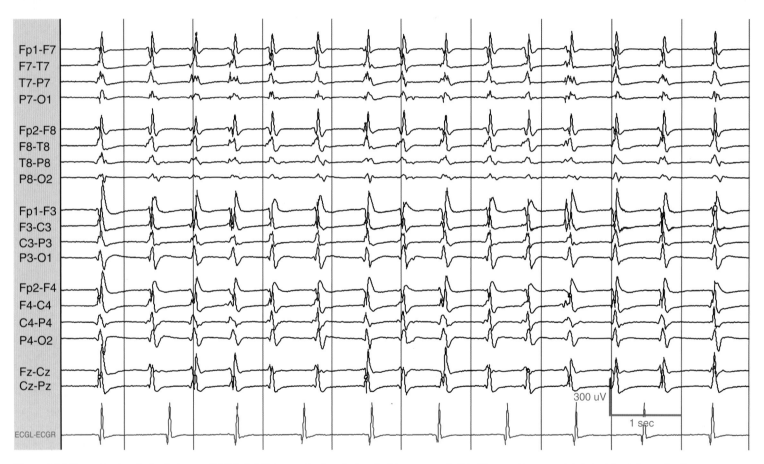

Figure 4-15 Generalized periodic discharges (GPDs). 1–2 Hz generalized periodic spike/sharp waves in this 45-year-old woman intubated for status epilepticus.

lag. GPDs are also often seen in relation to intermittent seizures and convulsive or nonconvulsive status epilepticus (see Chapter 6).

LATERALIZED PERIODIC DISCHARGES (LPDs)

LPDs (aka PLEDs; periodic lateralized epileptiform discharges) are repetitive discharges that occur at regular intervals maximally involving one hemisphere. The discharges may not be epileptiform and may consist, for example, of blunt delta waves that occur periodically (hence the letter "E" from PLEDs is out from the standardized ICU EEG nomenclature). LPDs are most commonly associated with an acute, structural lesion involving the cortex. Therefore, other findings of focal dysfunction such as focal slowing or attenuation are frequently accompanied in the ipsilateral hemisphere (Figure 4-16). The most common etiology of LPDs is ischemic stroke. Other frequent etiologies include viral encephalitis (particularly associated with, but not limited to herpes simplex virus, with frequent involvement of the temporal lobe), brain tumors, brain abscesses, and intracranial hemorrhages. LPDs may be seen without any obvious structural lesion. It is common to see LPDs in a location adjacent to the acute injury, presumably due to the relative inactivity of the severely damaged cortex. Bilateral independent PDs that are not synchronous are often caused by bilateral structural lesions (Figure 4-17).

Sometimes it is difficult to determine whether LPDs represent an ictal pattern or not, thus whether to treat LPDs or not. Often LPDs are simply a sign of dysfunction and do not represent seizures. If the patient is asymptomatic, no further treatment is indicated. In epilepsia partialis continua, focal clonic seizures can occur in a time-locked pattern to the contralateral LPDs. This clearly represents ongoing seizures. If the LPDs are greater than 3 Hz or if there is electrographic evolution, the pattern is considered ictal on electrographic criteria alone. Evolution is defined as at least 2 unequivocal, sequential changes in frequency, morphology, or location. However, the student may encounter situations that are not so clear. When there is no definite clinical correlation, look for other signs such as eye deviation, nystagmus, hemiparesis, sensory disturbances, aphasia, hemianopsia, or a depressed level of consciousness. In these cases treatment with AEDs should be considered, especially if there is not a structural lesion that clearly explains the neurological deficits. If clinical improvement along with improvement of LPDs is seen with a benzodiazepine or a loading dose of a fast-acting AED, it suggests that the pattern was ictal, and in this case further AED management is indicated.

FURTHER MODIFIERS OF RHYTHMIC AND PERIODIC PATTERNS

In an effort to standardize nomenclature, subtypes of PDs and RDA have been described on the basis of morphology. According to current ACNS nomenclature, they are called PDs + or RDA+ (Table 4-1). For PDs, the subtypes include superimposed fast activity (F) (Figure 4-18), rhythmic activity (R) (Figure 4-19), or both (FR). For RDA, the subtypes include superimposed fast activity (F) or spike/sharp waves (S) (Figure 4-20) or both (FS). Patterns of RDA + and PD + are considered to have a higher association with seizures than RDA or PD alone. The term SW connotes a pattern of spike and wave or sharp and wave and is used in patterns of spike/sharp and wave where there is no interval between one spike wave complex and the next (Figure 4-21). Of note, LPDs, rhythmic patterns, or even seizures can become activated with various stimuli (from clinical examinations, nursing care, noxious stimuli, environmental sounds, or spontaneous arousal, etc.) and this phenomena is described as stimulus-induced rhythmic, periodic, or ictal discharges (SIRPIDs) (Figure 4-22).

Text continued on p. 119

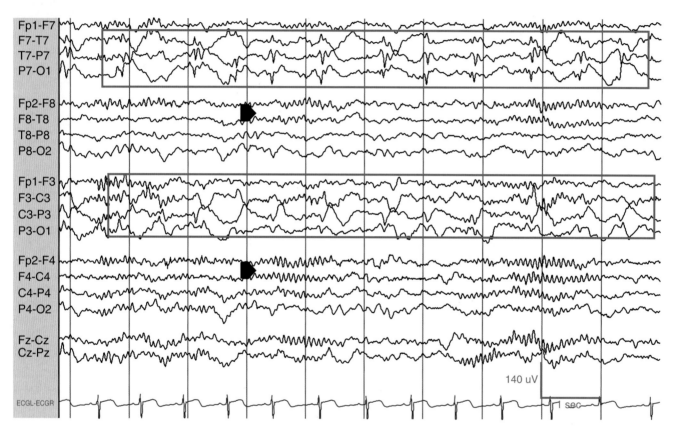

Figure 4-16 Lateralized periodic discharges (LPDs). A 9-year-old boy presented with headache, confusion, and right gaze deviation after an appendectomy. He was found to have a left transverse sinus venous thrombosis. EEG shows posteriorly predominant left hemisphere slowing and periodic spike waves occurring at 1 Hz (boxes). Additionally, notice that sleep spindles are seen better on the right (arrowhead).

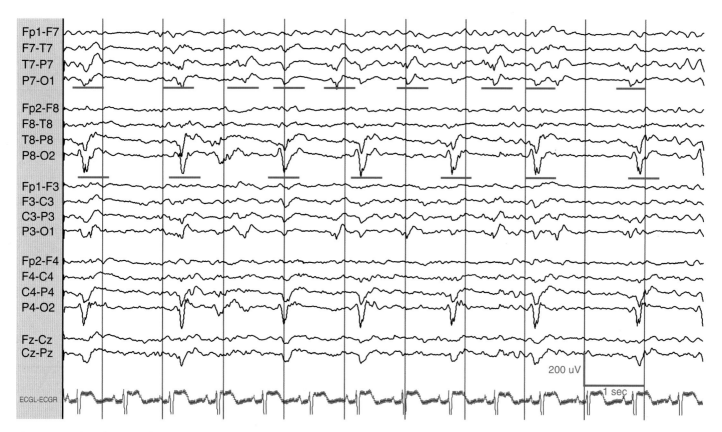

Figure 4-17 Bilateral independent periodic discharges (BIPDs). A 64-year-old woman with a history of a liver transplant presented with altered mental status and seizures. MRI brain revealed bilateral parieto-occipital T2 hyperintensities. EEG showed bilaterally independent (shown in underlines) periodic sharp waves/spike waves (BIPDs) that are more pronounced on the right.

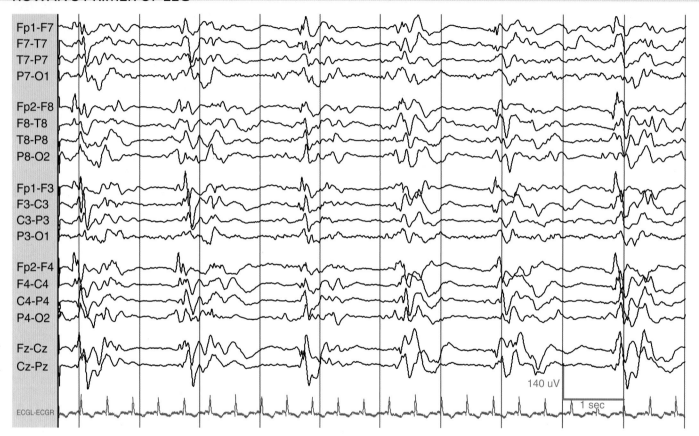

Figure 4-18 Generalized periodic discharges with superimposed fast activity (GPD+F). A 20-year-old woman with asthma presented with a severe asthma attack resulting in hypoxic-ischemic cerebral injury. EEG reveals generalized periodic spike/polyspike and wave discharges with superimposed fast frequencies (GPD+F) occurring every 1.5–2 seconds. In between the discharges, the background is diffusely attenuated.

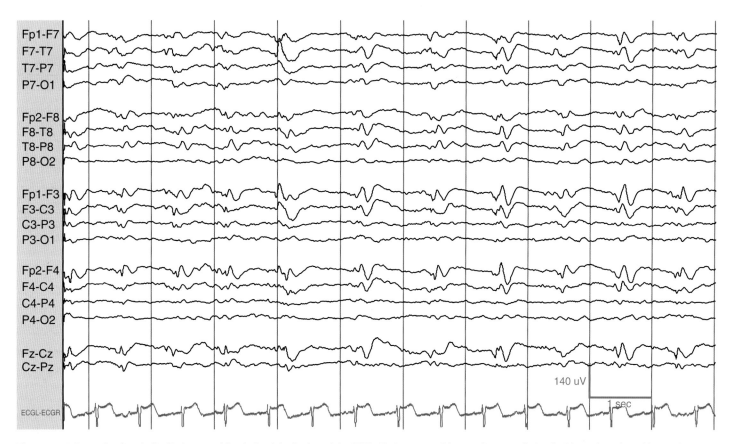

Figure 4-19 Generalized periodic discharges with admixed rhythmic activity (GPD+R). A 61-year-old man who was admitted with a subarachnoid hemorrhage. EEG revealed 1 Hz generalized periodic sharp waves with frequent admixed rhythmic delta activity (GPD+R) and an interval between complexes.

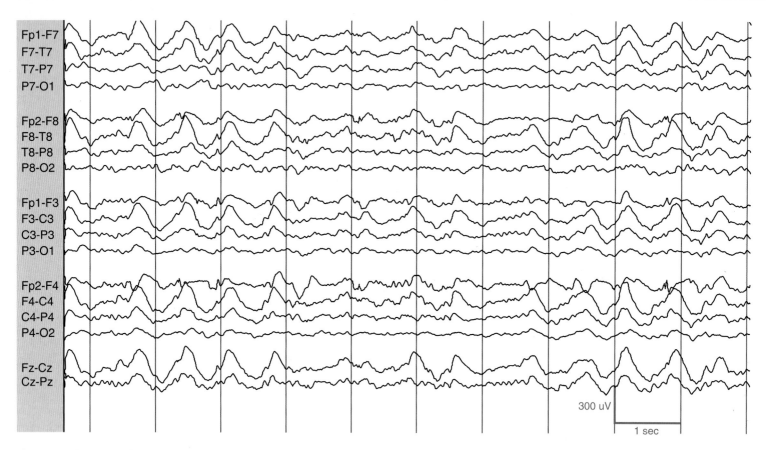

Figure 4-20 Generalized rhythmic delta activity with superimposed sharp waves or spikes (GRDA+S). A 14-year-old boy with autism and generalized epilepsy, presented with altered mental status after a witnessed seizure. EEG revealed frequent generalized rhythmic delta waves with superimposed spike waves (GRDA+S).

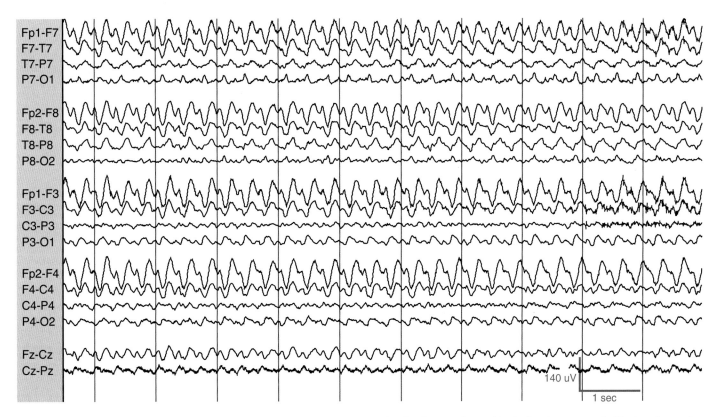

Figure 4-21 Generalized-spike and slow wave (GSW). A 29-year-old man with generalized epilepsy and a psychiatric disorder presented with altered mental status and decreased verbal output after an ECT treatment. EEG revealed continuous sharp and slow waves occurring at 2.5 Hz. An AED improved both the EEG and the patient's mental status. Though the frequency did not meet NCSE on the basis of electrographic criterion alone (not more than 3 Hz), combined with altered mental status and improvement after medication, this pattern represents NCSE.

117

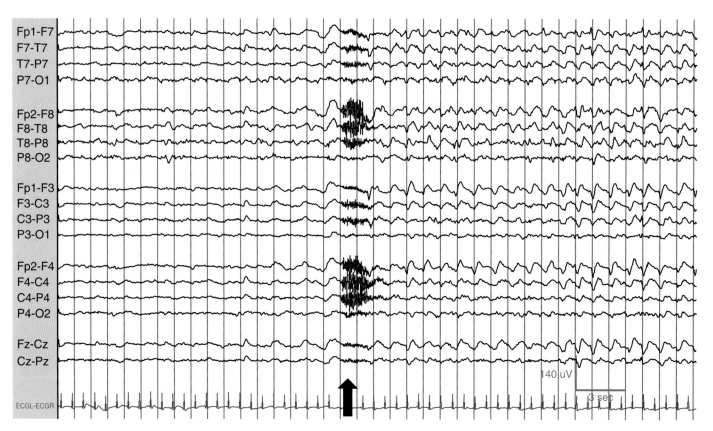

Figure 4-22 Stimulation-induced rhythmic, periodic, or ictal discharges (SIRPIDs). A 73-year-old woman with sepsis and respiratory failure. With a sternal rub (arrow), there is development of generalized rhythmic delta activity with admixed sharp waves (GRDA+S) at 1 Hz. This pattern was repeatedly seen with stimulation, and each lasted about a minute.

Further reading

Blume, W.T., Lemieux, J.F., 1988. Morphology of spikes in spike-and-wave complexes. Electroencephalogr. Clin. Neurophysiol. 69 (6), 508–515.

Chatrian, G.E., Shaw, C.M., Leffman, H., 1964. The Significance of Periodic Lateralized Epileptiform Discharges in EEG: An Electrographic, Clinical and Pathological Study. Electroencephalogr. Clin. Neurophysiol. 17, 177–193.

Garcia-Morales, I., Garcia, M.T., Galan-Davila, L., et al., 2002. Periodic lateralized epileptiform discharges: etiology, clinical aspects, seizures, and evolution in 130 patients. J. Clin. Neurophysiol. 19 (2), 172–177.

Gaspard, N., Manganas, L., Rampal, N., et al., 2013. Similarity of lateralized rhythmic delta activity to periodic lateralized epileptiform discharges in critically ill patients. JAMA Neurol. 70 (10), 1288–1295.

Gilmore, P.C., Brenner, R.P., 1981. Correlation of EEG, computerized tomography, and clinical findings. Study of 100 patients with focal delta activity. Arch. Neurol. 38 (6), 371–372.

Gloor, P., 1979. Generalized epilepsy with spike-and-wave discharge: a reinterpretation of its electrographic and clinical manifestations. The 1977 William G. Lennox Lecture, American Epilepsy Society. Epilepsia 20 (5), 571–588.

Gloor, P., Ball, G., Schaul, N., 1977. Brain lesions that produce delta waves in the EEG. Neurology 27 (4), 326–333.

Hirsch, L.J., Brenner, R.P., Drislane, F.W., et al., 2005. The ACNS subcommittee on research terminology for continuous EEG monitoring: proposed standardized terminology for rhythmic and periodic EEG patterns encountered in critically ill patients. J. Clin. Neurophysiol. 22 (2), 128–135.

Hirsch, L.J., Claassen, J., Mayer, S.A., et al., 2004. Stimulus-induced rhythmic, periodic, or ictal discharges (SIRPIDs): a common EEG phenomenon in the critically ill. Epilepsia 45 (2), 109–123.

Kuroiwa, Y., Celesia, G.G., 1980. Clinical significance of periodic EEG patterns. Arch. Neurol. 37 (1), 15–20.

Loiseau, P., Duche, B., 1989. Benign childhood epilepsy with centrotemporal spikes. Cleve. Clin. J. Med. 56 (Suppl. Pt 1), S17–S22, discussion S40–S42.

Ludwig, B.I., Marsan, C.A., 1975. Clinical ictal patterns in epileptic patients with occipital electroencephalographic foci. Neurology 25 (5), 463–471.

Marshall, D.W., Brey, R.L., Morse, M.W., 1988. Focal and/or lateralized polymorphic delta activity. Association with either "normal" or "nonfocal" computed tomographic scans. Arch. Neurol. 45 (1), 33–35.

Normand, M.M., Wszolek, Z.K., Klass, D.W., 1995. Temporal intermittent rhythmic delta activity in electroencephalograms. J. Clin. Neurophysiol. 12 (3), 280–284.

Pedley, T.A., Tharp, B.R., Herman, K., 1981. Clinical and electroencephalographic characteristics of midline parasagittal foci. Ann. Neurol. 9 (2), 142–149.

Pohlmann-Eden, B., Hoch, D.B., Cochius, J.I., et al., 1996. Periodic lateralized epileptiform discharges – a critical review. J. Clin. Neurophysiol. 13 (6), 519–530.

Pourmand, R.A., Markand, O.N., Thomas, C., 1984. Midline spike discharges: clinical and EEG correlates. Clin. Electroencephalogr. 15 (4), 232–236.

Reiher, J., Rivest, J., Grand'Maison, F., et al., 1991. Periodic lateralized epileptiform discharges with transitional rhythmic discharges: association with seizures. Electroencephalogr. Clin. Neurophysiol. 78 (1), 12–17.

Schaul, N., Gloor, P., Gotman, J., 1981. The EEG in deep midline lesions. Neurology 31 (2), 157–167.

Schaul, N., Lueders, H., Sachdev, K., 1981. Generalized, bilaterally synchronous bursts of slow waves in the EEG. Arch. Neurol. 38 (11), 690–692.

Westmoreland, B.F., Klass, D.W., Sharbrough, F.W., 1986. Chronic periodic lateralized epileptiform discharges. Arch. Neurol. 43 (5), 494–496.

Yoo, J.Y., Rampal, N., Petroff, O.A., et al., 2014. Brief potentially ictal rhythmic discharges in critically ill adults. JAMA Neurol. 71 (4), 454–462.

Zivin, L., Marsan, C.A., 1968. Incidence and prognostic significance of "epileptiform" activity in the eeg of non-epileptic subjects. Brain. J. Neurol. 91 (4), 751–778.

The EEG and epilepsy 5

When evaluating a new patient, the first line of inquiry for the clinician is, "is this a seizure?" There are many seizure mimics including parasomnias, syncope, transient ischemic attacks and psychogenic non-epileptic attacks (PNEA). A seizure is defined by the International League against Epilepsy (ILAE) to be "a transient occurrence of signs and/or symptoms due to abnormal excessive or synchronous neuronal activity in the brain." If the event in question is a seizure, the next line of inquiry is: Is the onset of the seizure generalized or focal? According to the ILAE generalized epileptic seizures begin at "some point within and rapidly engaging, bilaterally distributed networks. Such bilateral networks can include cortical and subcortical structures, but not necessarily include the entire cortex. Generalized seizures can be asymmetric." Focal epileptic seizures begin "within networks limited to one hemisphere. They may be discretely localized or more widely distributed." In some cases, there can be more than one seizure focus, which makes the epilepsy multifocal. Focal seizures can spread and involve both hemispheres, hence the type of epilepsy pertains to the onset and not the propagation pattern. The electrographic representation of a seizure is often similar between individuals (e.g., temporal lobe seizures from hippocampal sclerosis or an absence seizure). Electrographic seizures always disrupt the background, they generally evolve from faster frequencies to slower frequencies, and the shape of the waves (morphology) often changes over the course of the seizure, most commonly becoming higher in amplitude.

Multiple seizures from the same focus in the same individual will often have a very similar pattern. Table 5-1 delineates different seizure types and the EEG patterns associated with each seizure type.

The next question for discussion is whether or not an individual has epilepsy. Epilepsy is a disease of the brain defined by any of the following conditions: (1) At least two unprovoked (or reflex) seizures occurring >24 h apart; (2) one unprovoked (or reflex) seizure and a probability of further seizures similar to the general recurrence risk after two unprovoked seizures (at least 60%); and (3) diagnosis of an epilepsy syndrome. Of note, if an individual has a history of six seizures, all occurring in the setting of hypoglycemia from accidental insulin overuse, this individual does not have epilepsy. If a child has a single seizure, and the EEG is consistent with BECTS, by criteria #2 and 3, this child has epilepsy.

Following are brief discussions of nine important epilepsy syndromes along with the principal electrographic findings. An epilepsy syndrome or electroclinical syndrome specifically refers to identifiable disorders based upon multiple defining characteristics including but not limited to: age of onset, EEG characteristics, and seizure type. If the clinician is able to make an accurate diagnosis, the particular syndrome has implications for treatment, management, and prognosis. Table 5-2 provides a list of all the electroclinical syndromes and distinctive constellations as defined by the ILAE along with salient clinical and electrographic features.

Text continued on p. 143

Table 5-1 Seizure types and associated EEG patterns

	Clinical characteristics	EEG findings during the seizure
Generalized seizures		
Generalized tonic-clonic (GTC)	During the tonic phase, there is loss of consciousness and full body stiffening, often accompanied by a loud cry. In the clonic phase there is active rhythmic jerking.	Generalized fast activity (>10 Hz) that increases in amplitude and decreases in frequency during the tonic phase, with slow waves during the clonic phase (Figure 5-1).
Absence seizures		
Typical absence	Impairment of awareness for several seconds without loss of body tone. Sudden onset and cessation. Can have eyelid fluttering and eyes may drift upward. No post-ictal phase. Duration from 5–20 seconds.	Regular and symmetric generalized usually 3 Hz spike and slow wave complexes (Figure 4-6).
Atypical absence	Impairment of awareness often with insidious onsets and offsets. Can have an atonic component. Duration from 5–30 seconds.	Diffuse sometimes irregular spike and wave <2.5 Hz. Can be asymmetric.
Myoclonic absence	Rhythmic 2.5–4 Hz jerks, usually of the shoulders, arms, and legs during the absence seizure. Can have peri-oral jerks and an underlying tonic component. Duration is up to 60 seconds.	Regular and symmetric generalized 3 Hz spike and slow wave complexes.
Eyelid myoclonia	The first component is spasmodic 4–6 Hz blinking (eyelid myoclonia) often followed by mild impairment in consciousness. Seizures triggered with eye closure in the presence of light or with photic stimulation. Can have a subtle tonic component. Brief, each seizure lasts for seconds.	Generalized 3–6 Hz spike and polyspike and wave discharges that are triggered by eye closure or flickering light.
Myoclonic seizures		
Myoclonic	Brief (<100 ms), involuntary, shock-like, often irregular, jerking of the body. Can affect the whole body or just a part. Consciousness is typically not impaired.	Epileptic myoclonus is usually time locked to a generalized polyspike, which is followed by a wave. Myoclonus may not have an EEG correlate (Figures 5-2 and 5-3).
Myoclonic atonic	Brief myoclonic jerk followed by atonia (loss of muscle tone). Duration of myoclonic atonic seizure is 1–2 seconds.	Myoclonic jerk correlates with a generalized polyspike; atonia correlates with the after-going slow wave.
Myoclonic tonic	A myoclonic jerk or cluster of myoclonic jerks followed by a tonic seizure. Rare.	Myoclonic jerk correlates with a generalized spike, and tonic component may correlate with low-voltage fast activity.

Table 5-1 continued

	Clinical characteristics	EEG findings during the seizure
Tonic	Sudden onset of a rigid increase in muscle tone, often with stereotyped posturing of the limbs lasting from seconds to minutes. More frequent from sleep. Can be subtle (eye elevation) or massive. Autonomic features are common.	Low-voltage fast activity or 9–10 Hz activity, which may increase in amplitude and decrease in frequency (Figure 5-4).
Clonic	Generalized clonic seizures are rare consisting of LOC and bilateral 1–3 Hz rhythmic jerks with the jerk lasting for <100 ms. A clonic seizure differs from myoclonus in that it is rhythmic. Frequency diminishes but amplitude of jerk does not. Lasts from minutes to hours.	Fast activity >10 Hz or occasional spike and wave pattern.
Atonic	A sudden loss or decrease of muscle tone, which may be confined to a body part (head), or diffuse, leading to falls.	Electrodecrement, polyspike and wave, or low-amplitude fast activity.
Focal seizures		
Focal seizures	Seizure manifestation depends on the area of the brain that is seizing. People may be aware or have clouding of awareness. Symptoms and signs of focal seizures are numerous and varied and can include limb clonus, déjà vu, intense fear, or visual hallucinations. When there is clouding of the sensorium, people may have semi-purposeful picking movements known as automatisms. Focal seizures can spread and secondarily generalize leading to a generalized tonic clonic convulsion.	EEG can show rhythmic activity of varying morphologies from the brain region that is seizing (Figures 5-5, 5-6, and 5-7). In seizures that do not recruit at least 6 cm^2 of cortex, the EEG may show no change from the background on a scalp (not intracranial) recording.
Unknown		
Epileptic spasm	Onset of this seizure type is typically before age 1 year. Spasms are brief massive contractions of the axial muscles and can be clinically described as extensor, flexor, or mixed. In a mixed spasm there may be extension of the legs, abduction of the arms, and flexion of the neck. Spasms cluster around sleep transitions. Movement is usually symmetric. Consistent asymmetry implies a possible focal lesion.	The background EEG shows a high-voltage chaotic pattern known as hypsarrythmia. The EEG during a spasm can demonstrate a diffuse slow wave followed by electrodecrement, electrodecrement alone, or generalized paroxysmal low-amplitude fast activity (GPFA) (Figure 5-8).

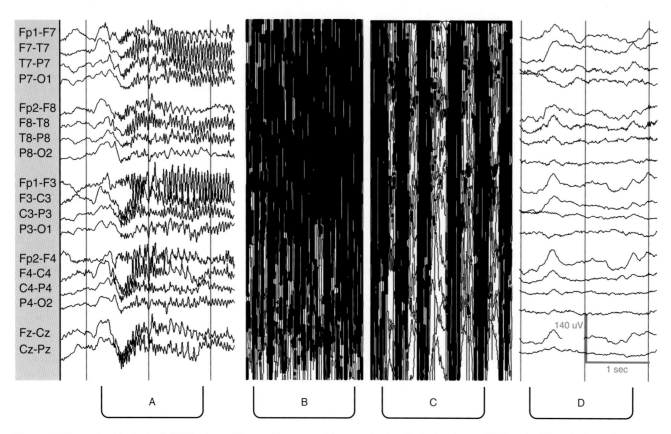

Figure 5-1 Generalized tonic clonic (GTC) seizure. 27-year-old woman with generalized tonic clonic seizures. (**A**) There is diffuse rhythmic fast activity at the seizure onset. (**B**) The patient becomes tonic, and the EEG is entirely obscured by muscle artifact. (**C**) Clonic activity follows with characteristic rhythmic muscle artifact. (**D**) After the seizure, there is postictal slowing. The entire seizure lasted 64 seconds.

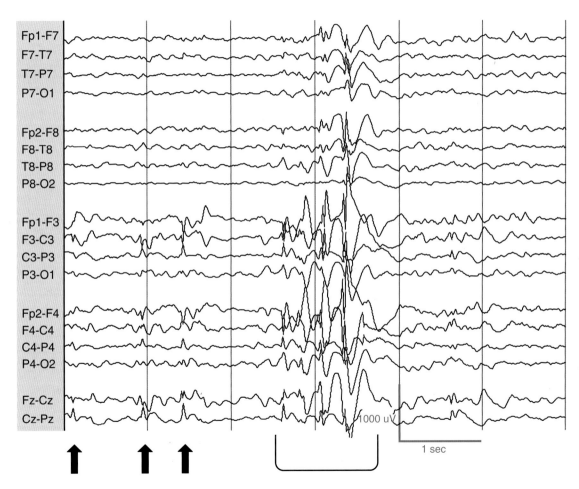

Figure 5-2 Myoclonic epilepsy of infancy. 4-year-old boy with myoclonus since 8 months of age. A bilateral synchronous burst of high-amplitude 4 Hz polyspike and wave (bracket) is more prominent in the parasagittal region for 0.5 sec and then becomes diffuse. A subtle myoclonic shoulder jerk was captured 100 msec after the last spike. Arrows show sporadic spikes, maximal in the parasagittal chain.

125

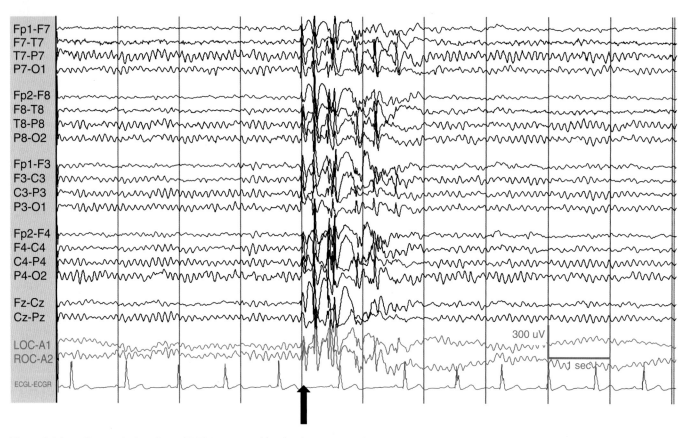

Figure 5-3 Juvenile myoclonic epilepsy (JME). A 17-year-old girl with JME. Generalized irregular 4 Hz spike and polyspike and wave (arrow) in the setting of a normal background. A jerk was reported by the technician during this discharge.

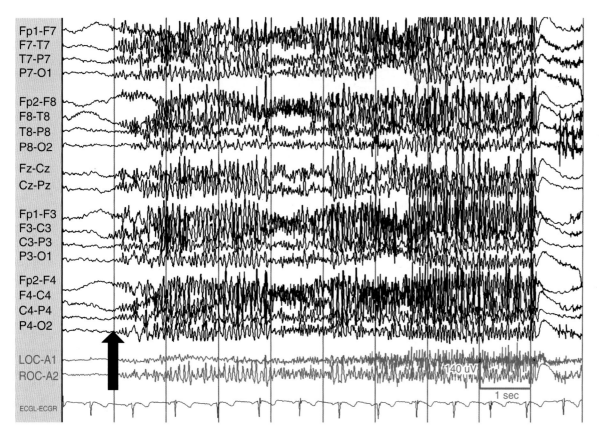

Figure 5-4 Tonic seizure. 56-year-old male with developmental delay and tonic seizures. Diffuse beta activity (arrow) and admixed EMG artifacts are present for 8 seconds. Clinically correlates with eye opening and subtle raising of his arms.

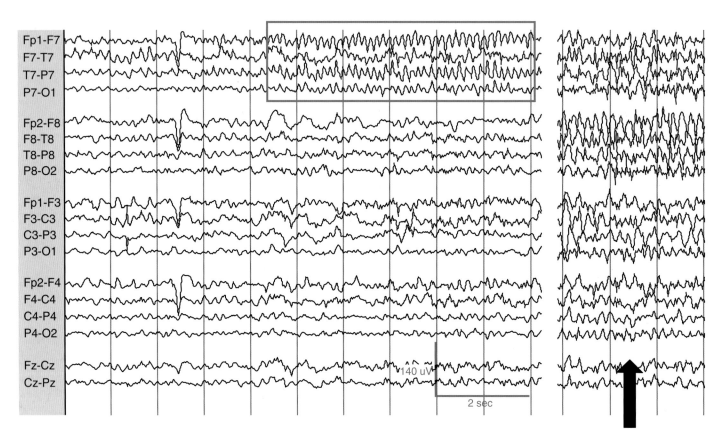

Figure 5-5 Mesial temporal lobe epilepsy (MTLE). Onset of a left temporal lobe seizure in a 58-year-old man with left MTS and schizophrenia. Rectangle shows rhythmic left temporal theta activity. After 30 seconds there is diffuse rhythmic activity of mixed frequencies (arrow).

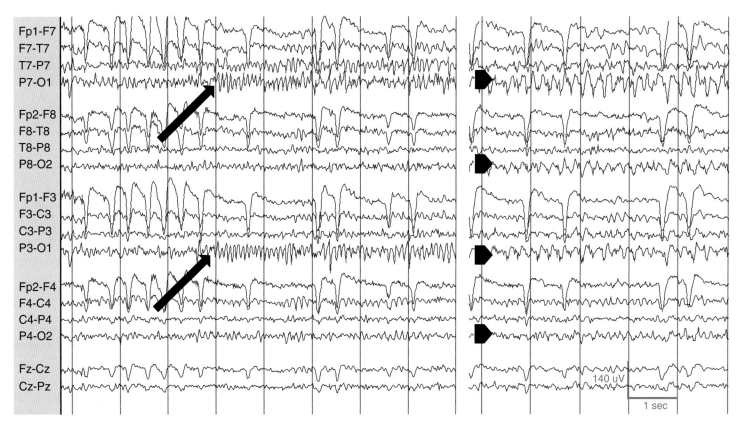

Figure 5-6 Occipital lobe seizure. A 21-year-old girl with Sturge–Weber syndrome, a left-sided port wine stain, and left posterior leptomeningeal angiomatosis. Onset of her left occipital seizure (arrow) with rhythmic alpha (mimicking a well-organized PDR!) evolves into bilateral occipital theta activity (arrowhead) with admixed spikes. Patient reports seeing a rainbow at onset.

129

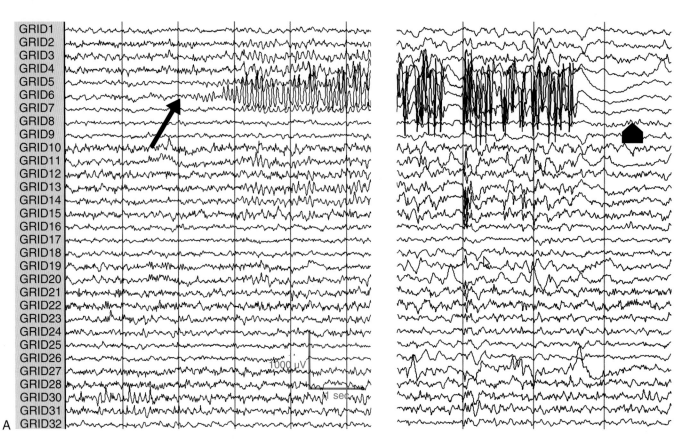

Figure 5-7 Frontal lobe epilepsy. (**A**) Intracranial recording of a right frontal seizure with a focal onset (arrow) in this 26-year-old man with refractory epilepsy. Clinically very bland with decreased responsiveness. Note postictal slowing (arrowhead).

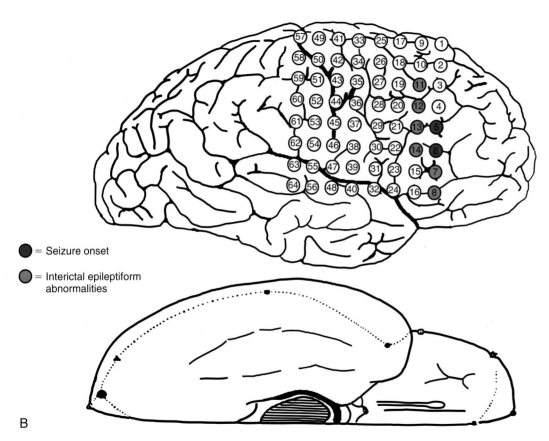

● = Seizure onset

● = Interictal epileptiform
    abnormalities

B

Figure 5-7, cont'd (B) Diagram of the 64 contact intracranial electrode grid used in this surgical case. Red indicates seizure onsets and green indicates a focus of interictal spikes or sharp waves. Epilepsy focus was resected and the patient has been seizure free since.

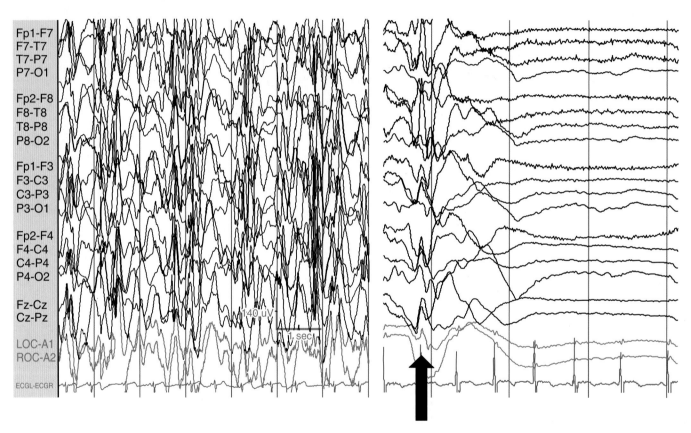

Figure 5-8 West syndrome. A 4-month-old previously normal baby boy with the development of infantile spasms. Hypsarrythmic background with high amplitude poorly organized chaotic appearing brain waves. A synchronous slow wave correlates with his clinical spasm (arrow) and is followed by electrodecrement.

Table 5-2 Electroclinical syndromes and other epilepsies

Syndrome Age of onset	Clinical	EEG
Neonatal period		
Benign familial neonatal epilepsy (BFNE) 3rd day of life	Usually clonic seizures, but can be apneic. Neurologically normal. Autosomal dominant. 10–15% progress to epilepsy. Multiple gene loci, usually a K^+ channel.	Normal background. Theta pointu alternant pattern (theta runs with admixed sharp waves) and multifocal spikes can be seen.
Early myoclonic encephalopathy (EME) Birth to several months	Stimulation-induced and spontaneous myoclonus and focal intractable seizures. Poor prognosis.	Burst suppression pattern. Myoclonus occurs during bursts.
Ohtahara syndrome Birth to several months	Tonic seizures, severe encephalopathy. Majority have severe structural abnormalities. Prognosis is poor. Can progress to IS and LGS.	Burst suppression pattern.
Infancy		
Epilepsy of infancy with migrating focal seizures <6 months	Unprovoked bilateral independent multifocal prolonged partial seizures that are intractable and followed by neurological deterioration. Infants are normal at onset.	Background normal at onset and then deteriorates. Multifocal spikes between seizures. Seizures with multifocal electrographic onsets.
West syndrome 3–12 months	Infantile spasms, developmental regression. Commonly progresses to LGS.	Hypsarrhythmic background. Diffuse slow or sharp wave with electrodecrement, electrodecrement alone or GPFA during a spasm (Figure 5-8).
Myoclonic epilepsy in infancy (MEI) 6 months–2 years	Myoclonic seizures, occasionally myoclonic atonic seizures. 30% have had febrile seizures. Most neurologically normal. Aggressive treatment is postulated to help with overall development. Remits by age 6.	Normal background. Myoclonus is associated with generalized spike and polyspike discharges (Figure 5-2).
Benign infantile epilepsy 3–10 months	Behavioral arrest, automatisms, can secondarily generalize. Remits by age 2.	Normal background. Can have vertex spikes in sleep.
Benign familial infantile epilepsy <1 year	Focal seizures, which may cluster. Easily controlled with medication. Neurologically normal. Autosomal dominant, usually Na^{2+} channel. Remits 1–2 years after onset.	Normal background.

Continued

Table 5-2 continued

Syndrome Age of onset	Clinical	EEG
Dravet syndrome <2 years, peak 6 months	Heat sensitive GTCC, hemiconvulsions, myoclonic seizures, atypical absence, ataxia, and neurological decline. Majority have SCN1A mutation.	Normal background at onset of disease, which worsens over time. Focal and generalized spikes interictally.
Myoclonic encephalopathy in nonprogressive disorders 1st day–5 years, peak 1 year	Repeated myoclonic status epilepticus. Focal, hemiclonic, GTCC can occur. Majority have an underlying genetic or structural disorder. Prognosis poor.	Background is slow with multifocal continuous spikes, sharp waves, or slow waves. Myoclonus may or may not correlate with a visible discharge.
Childhood		
Febrile seizures plus (FS+) (can start in infancy and continue past age 6)	Begins with febrile seizures. May have afebrile seizures of multiple types. Neurologically normal. Usually autosomal dominant.	Background normal. May have generalized spike and wave interictally.
Panayiotopoulos syndrome 2–8 years, peak 5 years	Rare nocturnal seizures with autonomic features and eye deviation. Often prolonged. Neurologically normal. Remits in 1–2 years.	Normal background. EEG variable with occipital, centrotemporal, parietal, and even generalized spikes. Discharges activate with sleep, eye closure, or darkness.
Epilepsy with myoclonic atonic (previously astatic) seizures 7 months–6 years, peak 2–6 years	Myoclonic atonic seizures, myoclonus, absence, GTCC, and tonic seizures. Neurologically normal at onset. Most have neurological deterioration. Prognosis is variable.	Background can be normal at onset. Interictal EEG can show generalized epileptiform potentials and parietal theta. Can go into status epilepticus after a GTCC (Figure 5-9).
Benign epilepsy with centrotemporal spikes (BECTS) 3–13 years, peak 7 years	Rare, usually nocturnal seizures with unilateral facial sensations and movements. Can generalize. Normal neurologically. Remits by age 16.	Normal background. Abundant bilateral or unilateral centrotemporal spikes activated by sleep (Figure 4-11).
Autosomal-dominant nocturnal frontal lobe epilepsy (ADNFLE) Variable, mean 9 years	Brief nocturnal frontal lobe seizures can be hypermotor or tonic. Neurologically normal. 30% refractory. Defects in nicotinic acetylcholine receptor subunit genes.	Normal background. May have anterior spikes. Seizures often are surface negative.
Late-onset childhood occipital epilepsy (Gastaut type) 3–16 years, peak 5 years	Frequent brief seizures with visual elementary hallucinations often with postictal migraine. Neurologically normal. 5% will develop recurrent epilepsy.	Mostly occipital spikes and sharp waves, activated by sleep, with eye closure or darkness (Figure 4-5).

Table 5-2 continued

Syndrome Age of onset	Clinical	EEG
Epilepsy with myoclonic absences 1–12 years, peak 7 years	Daily myoclonic absence seizures. GTCC, atonic, and absence seizures can be present. Usually neurologically normal. Cognitive function preserved with seizure control.	Background is normal. Interictal EEG with generalized 3 Hz spike and polyspike and wave.
Lennox–Gastaut syndrome (LGS) 1–7 years, peak 3–5 years	Multiple seizure types, including tonic (most common), myoclonic, GTCC, absence, atonic, and focal. Cognitive impairment. Refractory.	Background with slow spike and wave (1.5–2.5 Hz) (Figure 5-10). MISF and GPFA can be seen.
Epileptic encephalopathy with CSWS 2–12 years, peak 4–5 years	Neuropsychological and behavioral changes. Atypical absence, GTCC, atonic, and partial seizures. Refractory.	EEG shows CSWS with an anterior predominance (Figure 5-11).
Landau–Kleffner syndrome (LKS) 1–8 years, peak 3–5 years	Acquired aphasia presenting between 3 and 8 years. Seizures can occur and are usually easily controlled. Aphasia refractory.	EEG usually shows CSWS with a predominance in the temporal and temporal occipital area. Can have multifocal spikes.
Childhood absence epilepsy (CAE) 4–8 years, peak 5 years	Absence seizures. Neurologically normal. Majority will remit.	Normal background. Can have occipitally predominant rhythmic delta activity. Interictal generalized spikes or spike fragments. Seizures show 3 Hz spike and wave (Figure 4-6).
Adolescence–adult		
Juvenile absence epilepsy (JAE) 8–20 years, peak 9–13 years	Absence seizures, most with GTCC as well. Neurologically normal. Treatment is often lifelong.	Same as CAE (above).
Juvenile myoclonic epilepsy (JME) 8–25 years	Myoclonic seizures, often in the morning. Can have GTCC and absence. Neurologically normal. Easy to treat but usually requires lifelong medication.	Normal background. Interictally majority will have 4-6 Hz generalized polyspike and spike discharges (Figure 5-4).
Epilepsy with generalized tonic–clonic seizures alone 5–40 years, peak 11–23 years	GTCC within 1–2 hours of awakening. Neurologically normal. Usually requires lifelong treatment.	Normal background. Generalized spikes and polypsikes predominantly in sleep.

Continued

135

Table 5-2 continued

Syndrome / Age of onset	Clinical	EEG
Progressive myoclonic epilepsies (PME) Variable onset	Heterogenous group of disorders with myoclonus as a seizure type and typically a progressive and devastating course. (See Table 5-3 for more detail.)	Background may be normal at onset but worsens over time. Interictal EEG can show generalized and focal spikes (Figure 5-12). Large somatosensory or visual evoked potentials.
Autosomal dominant epilepsy with auditory features (ADEAF)	Focal seizures with buzzing, ringing or sudden inability to understand language. Neurologically normal. Can be a mutation in LGI1 gene. Responsive to treatment.	Background normal. Minority have focal temporal epileptiform potentials interictally. Ictal EEG shows temporal onset.
Other familial temporal lobe epilepsies	Temporal lobe seizures with a family history. Neurologically normal. Autosomal dominant.	Usually normal. Focal temporal lobe slowing can be seen. Rare temporal epileptiform potentials.
Less specific age relationship		
Familial focal epilepsy with variable foci (infancy to adult)	Each individual has a single focus, but family members may have different foci. Neurologically normal. Responsive to treatment. Autosomal dominant.	Normal background. May have focal epileptiform potentials interictally.
Reflex epilepsies	Syndrome in which *all* seizures are precipitated by sensory stimuli. Syndromes can involve multiple forms of photosensitivity, as well as reading, music, and startle. Can occur in neurologically normal and abnormal individuals.	These epilepsies can either be focal or generalized with either normal or abnormal backgrounds (Figure 2-10).
Distinctive constellations		
Mesial temporal lobe epilepsy with hippocampal sclerosis (MTLE with HS)	Typical auras include rising epigastric sensation, déjà vu or fear. Focal seizures with impaired awareness and automatisms. Neurologically normal individuals but some cognitive decline can occur with prolonged epilepsy. Often refractory to medical treatment.	Background may show focal slowing from involved temporal lobe. The majority have interictal anterior temporal sharp waves or spikes. Ictal EEG will often show rhythmic theta or alpha from the involved temporal lobe (Figure 5-5).
Rasmussen syndrome	EPC and other focal seizures. Progressive hemiplegia and cognitive decline. Hemispherectomy or hemispherotomy is the treatment of choice.	EEG shows focal slowing and epileptiform potentials on the affected side (Figure 5-13). EPC is often surface negative.

Table 5-2 continued

Syndrome Age of onset	Clinical	EEG
Gelastic seizures with hypothalamic hamartoma Variable, peak <12 months	Gelastic seizures are brief and frequent with bursts of laughing or giggling, can secondarily generalize. Neurologically normal at onset but at risk of deterioration.	Background normal at onset. Can worsen. Interictal spikes are rare and can be focal or generalized. Seizures are typically surface negative.
Hemiconvulsion–hemiplegia–epilepsy <2 years	Onset with a prolonged often febrile hemiconvulsion followed by flaccid hemiplegia, which does not entirely resolve. Subsequent refractory focal epilepsy with cognitive impairment. MRI shows edema followed by atrophy of involved hemisphere. Prognosis poor.	Focal slowing and epileptiform potentials on involved side.
Epilepsies that do not fit into any of the above diagnostic categories	These include epilepsies caused by malformations of cortical development, neurocutaneous syndromes, tumors, infections, trauma, angiomas, perinatal insults, strokes, and epilepsies of unknown cause.	EEG depends on particular cause. Seizures can be focal or generalized. Background can be normal or abnormal.
Conditions with epileptic seizures that are traditionally not diagnosed as a form per se		
Benign neonatal seizures (BNS) 5th day	Usually clonic seizures, but can be apneic. Neurologically normal. Seizures remit by 4–6 months of life.	Normal background. Theta pointu alternant pattern (theta runs with admixed sharp waves) and multifocal spikes can be seen.
Febrile seizures (FS) 3 months–5 years, peak 18–24 months	Seizures occurring in the setting of a high fever. Can be simple (<15 minutes, generalized) or complex (>15 minutes, focal, abnormal neurological examination and/or recurrent seizure within 24 hours). Family history common. Slight increased risk of developing epilepsy.	Background normal.

EPC, epilepsia partialis continua; GTCC, generalized tonic-clonic convulsion; GPFA, generalized paroxysmal fast activity; IS, infantile spasms; LGS, Lennox–Gastaut syndrome; MISF, multiple independent spike foci; CSWS, continuous spike and wave during sleep; SCN1A, alpha subunit of the neuronal type 1 sodium channel.

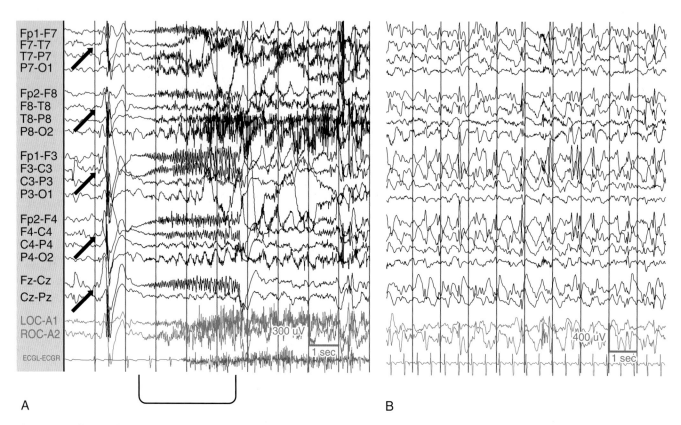

A   B

Figure 5-9 Epilepsy with myoclonic atonic seizure in a 7-year-old boy. (**A**) The EEG shows a generalized spike (arrows) followed by GPFA (bracket) and then rhythmic slowing and admixed muscle artifact. (**B**) After this seizure he became stuporous, drooling and ataxic. EEG consistent with a spike wave stupor (absence status epilepticus) with continuous high-amplitude 1–2 Hz spike and wave complexes. Mental status improved with very aggressive AED management.

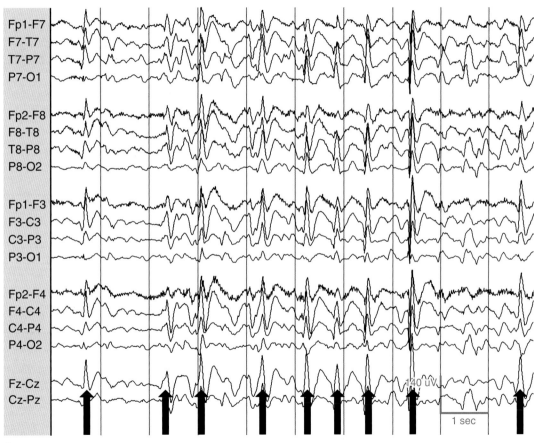

Figure 5-10 Lennox–Gastaut syndrome (LGS). (**A**) EEG shows frequent epochs with the characteristic slow 1.5–2 Hz spike and wave or sharp and wave (arrows) pattern in this 44-year-old with LGS. There was no clinical correlate with these discharges.

A

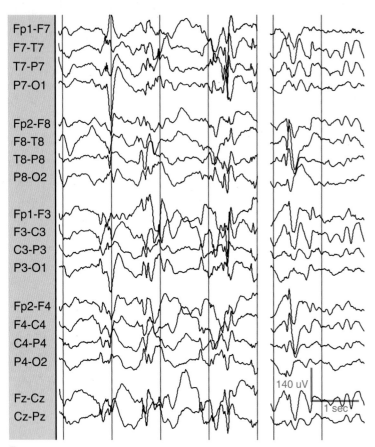

Figure 5-10, cont'd (**B**) Multiple independent spike foci (MISF) is another characteristic feature of LGS.

B

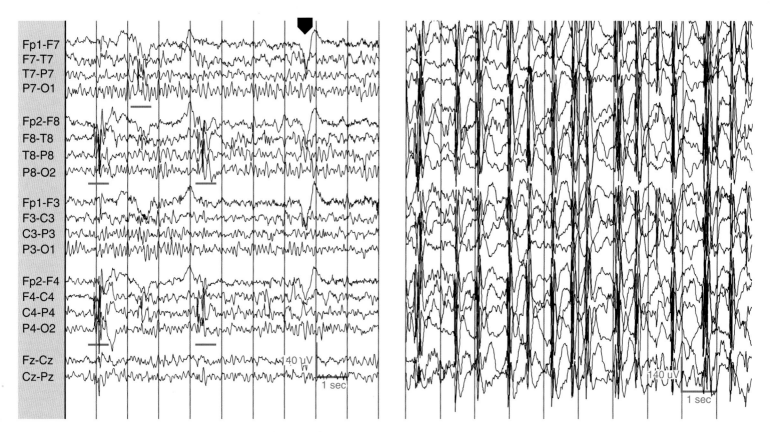

Figure 5-11 Epileptic encephalopathy with continuous spike wave of sleep (CSWS). Six-year-old girl who began to have behavioral problems in school, developmental regression, and rare seizures. (**A**) Occasional bilateral independent spikes and polyspikes (lines) during wakefulness. Eye blink (arrowhead) and a PDR of 8 Hz are seen. (**B**) CSWS with 1–2 Hz generalized spikes and polyspikes in sleep.

141

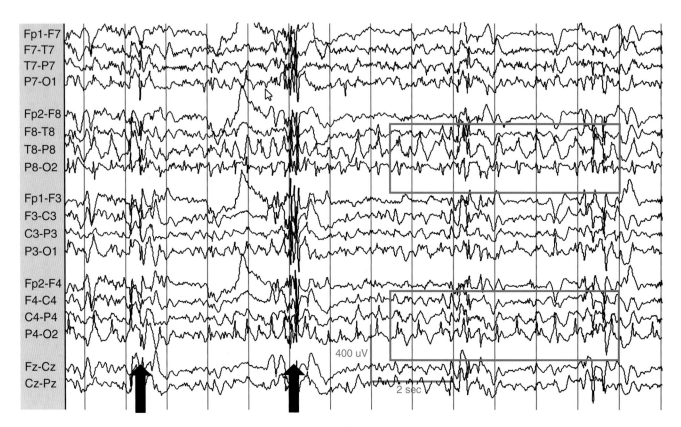

Figure 5-12 Progressive myoclonic epilepsy (Lafora's disease). 16-year-old boy originally diagnosed with JME because of the presence of generalized polyspikes (arrows), but upon closer inspection a number of features are inconsistent with JME including a suboptimally organized and slow background with right posterior 2 Hz spike and wave (rectangle).

142

West syndrome

This serious illness typically has its onset between 3 and 12 months, and nearly always before the age of 2 years. The typical spasm consists of a sudden, brief flexion movement of the body with flexion of the neck and abduction of the arms (so-called Salaam seizures). Extension of the neck and lower extremities may occur. The attacks are frequent, occurring in clusters around sleep transitions, and are associated with regression of milestones. Causes are multiple and include cerebral malformations (e.g., agyria, pachygyria), perinatal brain damage, tuberous sclerosis, and a variety of metabolic disorders (e.g., non-ketotic hyperglycinemia). In about 15% of cases, no underlying cause can be identified.

The typical EEG feature is hypsarrhythmia, a more or less continuous, high-voltage (>350 μV), chaotic, slow wave pattern with frequent multi-focal spikes and sharp waves (Figure 5-8). Variations of this background pattern, termed modified hypsarrhythmia, are common. These include a burst suppression pattern, focal features (i.e., hemi-hypsarrhythmia), or slow waves without spikes. During the spasm, the most common pattern is a diffuse high-amplitude slow or sharp wave followed by electrodecrement (Figure 5-8), but electrodecrement alone or low-amplitude fast activity can be seen. About half of the patients develop Lennox–Gastaut syndrome (LGS), and at least 80% develop cognitive impairment. Spasms are notoriously difficult to treat. Adrenocorticotropic hormone (ACTH) is highly effective and requires close monitoring due to the potential side effects of hypertension, cushinoid obesity, electrolyte disturbances, cardiomyopathy, or immunosuppression. Vigabatrin is another effective medication for spasms, particularly in children with tuberous sclerosis.

Dravet's syndrome (severe myoclonic epilepsy of infancy)

Infants present with febrile seizures before the age of 2, typically around 6 months. Hot baths, infection, fever, and strong emotion can all trigger seizures. After several months, afebrile convulsions occur followed by the development of myoclonic (onset 1–5 years) and atypical absence seizures. Hemiconvulsions with unilateral clonic activity are characteristic at the onset of the disease but less common in children older than the age of 3. Obtunded states with spike and wave and rare tonic seizures can be present. The infants may be normal at onset but suffer from developmental delay and ataxia as the disease progresses. The EEG background is usually normal at onset and deteriorates over time. Interictally, there can be generalized and focal epileptiform potentials. The disease is associated in the majority of cases with a mutation in alpha subunit of the neuronal type 1 sodium channel (SCN1A). Due to the abundance of this channel on the inhibitory interneurons, any AEDs that act on the sodium channel (including phenytoin, carbamazepine and lamotrigine) can make the seizures worse and even propel the individual into status epilepticus. Agents should be chosen which are broad spectrum AND not sodium channel blockers. The severity of the seizures correlates with the severity of neurological decline and about 90% of children with Dravet are medically refractory. Recently medical marijuana, specifically cannabidiol, is being investigated in the treatment of Dravet as well as LGS.

Benign epilepsy with centrotemporal spikes (BECTS)

This common epilepsy syndrome is easily recognized and also commonly referred to as benign rolandic epilepsy. Onset is between the ages of 3 and 13, and the disorder always remits by age 16. Imaging studies are normal. The neurological examination is normal, as is the EEG background (well-organized with no focal or generalized slowing). There may be a family history.

Common features during seizures include vocalization with guttural sounds, hypersalivation, unilateral oral/facial sensations, and clenching of the teeth. There may be hemifacial movements, hemiconvulsions, and even generalized tonic-clonic convulsions. Seizures typically occur upon falling asleep or upon awakening. Seizures are usually rare in BECTS but a small minority may have frequent events. Subtle neuro-psychological difficulties have been encountered in children with BECTS, typically involving attention and reading. These difficulties are thought to resolve when the interictal EEG improves in mid adolescence.

Epileptiform discharges consist of sharp waves and/or spikes, often biphasic in configuration, occurring in the centrotemporal regions (C3/T3 and/or C4/T4) (Figure 4-9). The discharges may occur in wakefulness but are usually markedly activated by drowsiness and sleep. Isolated sharp waves while awake often transform into grouped or rhythmic discharges during sleep and often alternate between the two hemispheres. There may be a left or right preponderance. Strictly unilateral discharges may also be seen. Rarely, some patients will have generalized discharges as well. Note that the EEG may contain many discharges, although few seizures have ever occurred. Interestingly, these discharges are seen in nearly 1% of children without a seizure disorder and it is estimated that only about 10% of children with centrotemporal sharp waves and spikes go on to develop epilepsy.

There is no universal agreement on treatment. Considering the benign nature of the condition, the debate is whether to treat or not. If treatment is elected, the best therapy may be one that reduces interictal discharges as well as seizures (e.g., levetiracetam, valproic acid).

Lennox–gastaut syndrome (LGS)

LGS has its onset in early childhood, usually around 3–5 years. The classic triad of LGS is cognitive impairment, multiple seizure types, and slow spike and wave (1.5–2.5 Hz) on the EEG. Seizure types include tonic (most common), atonic, myoclonic, focal seizures, and atypical absence. Status epilepticus is not rare and occurs in at least 50% of LGS patients. Typically it is non-convulsive with atypical absence stupor and tonic seizures admixed.

About one-third of cases of LGS are of unknown cause, the remainder being due to congenital malformations, tuberous sclerosis, encephalitis, and perinatal hypoxic brain damage. Infants can first develop West syndrome in infancy and later evolve into LGS.

The EEG typically demonstrates a pattern of generalized slow spike-wave discharges at an average of 2 Hz (Figure 5-10). In addition, multiple independent spike foci (MISF) and generalized paroxysmal fast activity (GPFA) are common.

Treatment of the seizures is difficult. ACTH, the ketogenic diet, multiple AEDs, vagal nerve stimulator, and corpus callosotomy have all been used with variable success. As the clinician struggles to control the seizures, overmedication can occur, which can worsen mentation and balance.

Prognosis is generally poor, and the majority suffer from severe cognitive impairment, even if the seizures are eventually controlled.

Childhood absence epilepsy (CAE)

CAE usually makes its appearance at the time the child enters school at about age 5 years, with a range between 4 and 8 years. These children are essentially normal though with higher rates of attentional difficulties. The attacks themselves consist of staring episodes, with or without eye blinking, and generally are not longer than 10 seconds in duration. Minor automatisms appear in about 30% of cases, and occasional clonic or tonic features may be observed. Hyperventilation increases the likelihood of seizure occurrence, and pediatric neurologists routinely carry out the procedure in their offices in suspected cases. In the untreated state, hundreds of seizures may occur in a single day. There often is a family history of absence seizures, and twin studies have demonstrated a 75–80% concordance for the seizures and the EEG trait.

The EEG is characteristic, demonstrating generalized 3 Hz spike and wave discharges (Figure 4-6). During the seizure the child is unresponsive but recovers immediately upon discharge cessation. At the same time the normal background rhythms are restored without evidence of postictal slowing. The background is typically normal in between discharges. However, bursts of occipitally predominant rhythmic delta activity are not uncommon. During sleep there is distortion of the generalized discharges – the frequency band declines, and polyspike-wave complexes are not uncommon.

A number of AEDs including ethosuximide, valproate, lamotrigine, and topiramate are likely to lead to complete seizure suppression. Agents used for focal epilepsy like carbamazepine and phenytoin can worsen CAE. Numbers vary widely throughout the literature and 57–74% of children with CAE will have a complete remission of their epilepsy in adolescence. If absence seizures are the only seizure type, about 80% of children will remit. If a child with absence seizures has a GTCC, the rate of remission is only 30%. Early institution of therapy improves outcome. Of note, if a child with CAE is treated with ethosuximide and has a GTCC, another agent must be added. Ethosuximide is a great medication for absence seizures but does not control generalized convulsions.

Juvenile myoclonic epilepsy (JME)

Patients with JME are typically adolescents who are neurologically normal with normal imaging. The first GTCC seizure often occurs after a night of poor sleep and/or alcohol intake. There is frequently a history of myoclonic jerks in the morning, which may be bilateral or unilateral. Adolescents may just feel that they are clumsy in the morning and frequently drop spoons or fling their toothbrush. A series of myoclonic jerks can lead to a GTCC seizure. Absence seizures are seen in a substantial minority. There is a genetic predisposition. The interictal EEG demonstrates 4–6 Hz generalized spike and polyspike-wave discharges (Figure 5-4). Thirty to 50% of patients with JME are photosensitive and their EEG will show generalized spikes or polyspikes with photic

stimulation. The seizures are usually well controlled with a broad-spectrum AED. Limiting alcohol consumption and achieving regular sleep are cornerstones of therapy.

A particular feature of the syndrome should be emphasized: Treatment is continued indefinitely, as relapse after discontinuation of AEDs occurs in the majority of patients.

Progressive myoclonic epilepsies (PME)

PMEs are a rare and heterogeneous group of disorders that are classified together because of their progressive and refractory nature and because myoclonus is one of the main seizure types. There is no cure for any of these disorders, and the diagnosis is devastating. Onset is typically in late childhood or early adolescence. In the beginning, the background EEG is typically normal with sporadic generalized spike and polyspike discharges. The initial diagnosis may erroneously be JME. Over time, the background becomes slower and less organized. Individuals with PME have large somatosensory evoked potentials and visual evoked potentials, indicating the overall lack of inhibition to stimulation. Photosensitivity is common. Treatment is with any broad-spectrum AED that is efficacious against myoclonus: valproic acid, benzodiazepines, levetiracetam, topiramate, and zonisamide either alone or in combination are all reasonable choices. Ketogenic diet has been tried as well. Clinical and electrographic features of the most common diseases in this category can be found in Table 5-3.

Mesial temporal lobe epilepsy with hippocampal sclerosis (MTLE with HS)

HS accounts for about 20% of all adult epilepsy. MTLE typically causes focal seizures with an aura. The aura can be nausea, a rising epigastric sensation, intense fear, déjà vu, or an olfactory hallucination. This aura can pass after a few seconds to minutes or it can develop into a seizure

Table 5-3 Progressive myoclonic epilepsy

PME	Disease characteristics
Unverricht–Lundborg disease (Baltic myoclonus)	Stimulus-sensitive myoclonus, GTCC, ataxia, and tremor. Cognition is relatively spared. Recessive mutation in EPM1. Most common PME.
Lafora's disease	Stimulus-sensitive myoclonus, progressive mental decline, visual seizures, atonic seizures, GTCC and blindness. EEG often has occipital spikes and occipital seizures, which is a distinguishing feature (Figure 5-7). Recessive mutations in either EPM2A (60%) or EPM2B (35%) causing a polyglucosan storage disorder.
Myoclonic epilepsy with ragged red fibers (MERRF)	Mitochondrial disorder characterized by myoclonus, generalized epilepsy, and ataxia. Can have myopathy, diabetes, deafness, cognitive decline, external ophthalmoplegia, and neuropathy. MRI may show cortical atrophy and low signal in basal ganglia. May be sporadic or autosomally inherited. Muscle biopsy shows ragged red fibers in vast majority.
Neuronal ceroid lipofuscinoses (NCL)	Multiple disease subtypes. Most frequent age of onset is 4–7. Children develop visual loss, GTCC, subtle myoclonus, psychiatric features, and later dementia. Death within 10 years of diagnosis is common. Autosomal recessive disorder with different genes depending on subtype all causing abnormal amounts of lipopigments in lysosomes. MRI is abnormal.
Sialidoses type 1	GTCC and an intention tremor begin in adolescence or adulthood. Cognitive decline, spasticity, ataxia, and a painful neuropathy can all occur. May have a cherry red spot on examination of fundus. Autosomal recessive disorder caused by deficiency of neuraminidase A.
Dentato-rubro-pallido-luysian atrophy (DRPLA)	Clinical features include epilepsy, Parkinsonism, chorea, athetosis, myoclonus, and dementia. Frequently photosensitive. Rare autosomal dominant triplicate repeat disorder.

with impairment of awareness. At this stage, the eyes remain open but the individual is not responding properly and there may be automatisms of chewing or picking movements. Autonomic features are common with sweating, pupillary dilatation and heart rate changes. A secondarily generalized seizure can occur. Seizures with impaired awareness are often followed by fatigue and confusion.

The interictal EEG in 90% of patients will show sporadic sharp waves and spikes from the affected side, often with phase reversal at the F7 (left) or F8 (right) electrodes. There may be some associated, intermittent, and often subtle temporal lobe slowing. The most common ictal pattern is rhythmic temporal theta or alpha activity within 30 seconds of symptom onset (Figure 5-5). There may be some ipsilateral postictal slowing.

146

The etiology is not delineated in the majority of cases of HS, but febrile seizures, particularly prolonged, and status epilepticus are possibly causative in some cases as is antecedent traumatic brain injury.

Medication is the first-line treatment for MTLE with HS, but the clinician should be aware that 90% of patients with this condition will be pharmaco-resistant. Refractory patients should be considered for surgical treatment. The majority of patients with refractory MTLE with HS will be free of disabling seizures after surgery and have a better quality of life.

Rasmussen's encephalitis

This is a rare epilepsy syndrome, which in the vast majority of cases presents in childhood. A typical case would start with the development of partial seizures (with or without secondary generalization) in an otherwise healthy child between the ages of 1 and 13. Status epilepticus is not an uncommon first manifestation. Epilepsia partialis continua (EPC), ongoing focal clonic motor seizures without impairment of consciousness, is a hallmark of the entity. As the disease develops, there is a progressive hemiparesis and cognitive decline. MRI early in the disorder may show focal hyperintense signal in the cortex of the affected side on T2 or FLAIR sequences. Later there is progressive hemi-atrophy. Multiple auto-antibodies have been implicated, including anti-GluR3 and the neuronal acetylcholine receptor alpha 7 subunit. However, these are neither sensitive nor specific. The EEG may show focal slowing in the abnormal hemisphere, as well as multifocal, usually but not always lateralized epileptiform potentials (Figure 5-13). EPC often has no electrographic correlate. Rasmussen's is difficult if not impossible to treat with AEDs. Surgical resection and/or disconnection (hemispherectomy/ hemispherotomy) of the affected side is essentially the only effective treatment for this disorder. The vast majority of children (>90%) who underwent this procedure were rendered free of disabling seizures with the majority being entirely seizure free.

THE VALUE OF THE EEG IN EPILEPSY PROGNOSIS

Many clinicians place great value on the EEG when deciding whether or not to discontinue AEDs in seizure-free patients. Although it seems obvious that an epileptiform EEG should stay one's hand from discontinuing AEDs, the correlation between potential seizure recurrence and the presence of discharges is not consistent. Many studies have been published, with varying results. A benchmark for considering discontinuation is 2 years of seizure freedom, although this varies from 2–5 years depending on the particular study.

In adults, a good rule of thumb is that the patient, after 2 years of seizure freedom, has a 60% chance of remaining seizure free after slow withdrawal of medication. The lack of epileptiform activity on the EEG means a better chance of success, but this by no means is a guarantee. Ongoing either generalized or focal spikes decrease the rate of success. If patients with generalized epilepsy continue to display generalized spike-wave discharges, the probability of seizure recurrence is relatively high. Note that even brief discharges of 1–2 seconds' duration are likely to correlate with very brief clinical lapses of which the patient is unaware. In this case, medication should be continued.

Multiple clinical circumstances increase the rate of relapse including a diagnosis of JME or post-traumatic epilepsy, multiple seizures prior to control with AEDs, tonic clonic seizures, polytherapy, and an abnormal neurological examination.

Other considerations are important, e.g., the patient's temperament and his or her occupation (is driving required?). The issue must be discussed in detail with the patient, offering the pros and cons of discontinuation. Some patients do not want to take AEDs if not absolutely

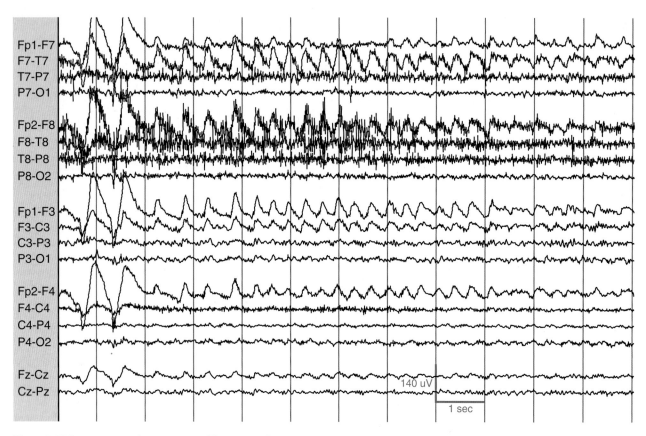

Figure 5-13 Rasmussen syndrome. 30-year-old woman with Rasmussen's encephalitis who is status post an incomplete functional hemispherotomy on the right. EEG shows attenuation of faster frequencies on the right and left anterior lateralized rhythmic delta activity (LRDA) with some reflection on the right, which correlates with behavioral arrest and is thus a seizure.

148

necessary and are willing to chance the possibility of seizure recurrence. Others are quite fearful of a possible seizure and are adamant about remaining on AEDs. As with all physician–patient interactions, a mutual understanding is essential for arriving at an individualized plan that is acceptable to both parties. The situation is different in children, and there is a good chance of "growing out of" some of the childhood onset epilepsies.

REFRACTORY EPILEPSY

Despite the development of numerous new AEDs, about 30% of patients are medically refractory, meaning that they continue to have seizures despite appropriately chosen medication. In these cases, surgical intervention should be considered. If the patient, through extensive testing, is deemed to be a surgical candidate but the focus has not been adequately localized with extra-cranial EEG, intracranial electrodes can be placed over the region of suspected onset (Figure 5-14A). The patient then returns to the intensive care unit or epilepsy monitory unit with intracranial electrodes, and medications are lowered to induce seizures (Figure 5-7). The same principles of reading EEGs apply to intracranial EEGs. The difference is that usual landmarks of the normal EEG like PDR, sleep spindles, and vertex waves are not usually seen intracranially. If the seizures are localized, the next question is, can the focus be removed without causing a neurological deficit? One technique used to answer that question is brain mapping. During brain mapping, the intracranial electrodes are stimulated in pairs to precisely delineate motor, sensory, language, and visual areas (Figure 5-14B). The hope is that the seizure focus is not overlying eloquent cortex and can be safely resected.

A comprehensive discussion of the possible treatments of refractory epilepsy is outside the scope of this primer. However, one new technique deserves special mention, as it uses ongoing EEG data to treat refractory epilepsy. Responsive neurostimulation (RNS) is a technique that can be considered for focal epilepsy, which is refractory but not amenable to surgical resection. This occurs if the epilepsy focus is over eloquent cortex or if there are more than one foci. Electrodes are placed intracranially with either strips laying over the surface of the brain or depths within the brain. These electrodes are programmed to detect the onset

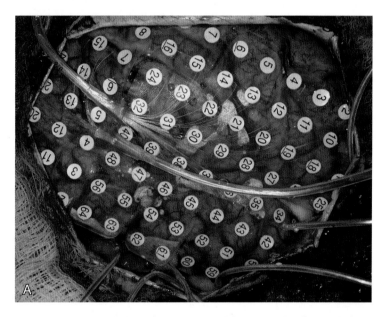

Figure 5-14 Intracranial electrodes. (**A**) 61-year-old woman with refractory epilepsy after a stroke with intracranial electrodes placed over the frontal, parietal, and temporal lobe on the right.

Continued

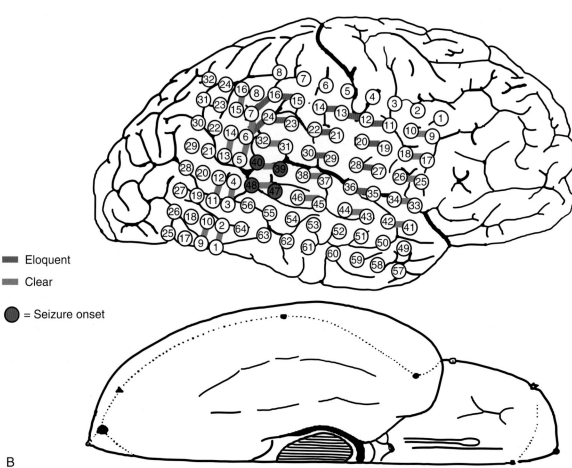

Eloquent

Clear

= Seizure onset

Figure 5-14, cont'd(B) Seizure onsets were found to be coming from electrodes 39–40 and 47–48 primarily. When these areas were stimulated during brain mapping, there was no effect to the patient and they were determined to be clear (green). If stimulating an area had an effect, it was marked purple on the diagram, and the exact effect was detailed in a separate report. Hence, the seizure focus was close to eloquent cortex but not overlying it and the epilepsy focus was resected. During brain mapping, stimulation can cause an increase in spikes and sharp waves (after discharges) or a frank electrographic seizure. Frank seizures can be aborted by rapid trains of stimulation.

B

of a possible seizure and then stimulate the brain to stop the seizure from developing. Detection and stimulation parameters are adjusted over time so that the best result can be obtained for each individual (Figure 5-15). The RNS device has the added benefit of providing ongoing EEG data to the epileptologist, which can be very useful as many patients are not aware of when they are having seizures.

THE EEG IN SEIZURE MIMICS

When seizures are possibly but not definitely the etiology of an event, the EEG is an indispensable tool in making an accurate diagnosis. Common seizure mimics in sleep are night terrors and somnambulism, both of which occur in slow wave sleep. In adults, REM behavior disorder, with loss of the normal paralysis in REM sleep, leads to acting out of dreams. The EEG shows REM sleep and the events that can be hyperkinetic are not particularly stereotyped. During breath-holding spells in children and in syncope in all ages, the EEG will show diffuse slowing but no underlying seizure activity (Figure 5-16). Movement disorders, self-stimulatory behavior, confusional migraines, transient ischemic attacks, benign myoclonus of sleep, daydreaming, cataplexy, narcolepsy, and reflux (in infants) can all mimic seizures. For all of these, the EEG shows no underlying seizure.

The most frequently encountered mimic in the epilepsy monitoring unit is psychogenic non-epileptic attacks (PNEA). It is essential to capture the event in question with VEEG to make the diagnosis, as a normal EEG background is often seen in epilepsy. In addition, a significant minority of patients (percentages vary widely but approximately 10–19%) will have both PNEA and epilepsy. The same individual may have interictal spikes and events that are psychogenic. Any individual

with events that are not controlled with AEDs should be brought in for EEG monitoring because the diagnosis has a profound impact on the approach to care: The events may be uncontrolled because the epilepsy is refractory, and a more aggressive approach is needed or the events may be uncontrolled because the diagnosis is PNEA and in this case no AEDs are needed. Given the overlap between epilepsy and PNEA, it is important to capture all known clinical events before discharging the patient off AEDs. The authors suggest both referral to psychiatry and continued neurological follow-up of patients with PNEA. The neurological follow-up is to help reinforce the diagnosis of PNEA and to prevent the re-accumulation of unnecessary and potentially harmful AEDs from other well-meaning but misinformed physicians.

PNEA have some clinical characteristics that may be helpful: asynchronous shaking, pelvic thrusting, erratic stopping and starting of movements with various amplitudes and frequencies, eyes closed, head shaking from side to side, and bilateral movements with preserved consciousness. While the EEG is often obscured during PNEA by movement, if there are brief pauses, a normal PDR can be discerned. There is no postictal slowing after an event.

Beware, surface negative seizures in which the seizure activity is either too small (<6 cm^2 of activated cortex) or too distant from the recording electrodes can be mistaken for PNEA. For example, EPC with ongoing focal motor activity is surface negative about 50% of the time. The movement is not suppressible and will often persist in sleep, which is the key to diagnosis. Frontal seizures, which can be bizarre and hyperkinetic, are often surface negative. These tend to be brief and highly stereotyped. When an event shows no EEG correlate, the video is not trivial as the clinician must rely on a thorough knowledge of seizure semiology in order to make the right diagnosis.

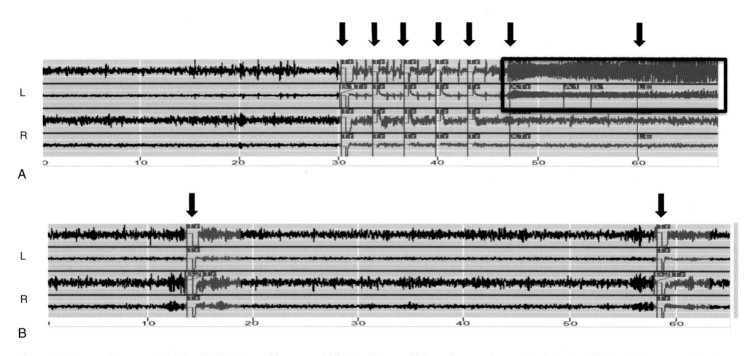

Figure 5-15 Responsive neurostimulation (RNS). 55-year-old woman with bilateral temporal lobe epilepsy underwent implantation of bilateral hippocampal depth electrodes in the RNS system. Compressed EEG data from the left (L) and right (R) hippocampi. (**A**) The blue shows the detection onset of a possible seizure with multiple stimulation (arrows) delivered to stop the seizure. The stimulation fails and a clear left temporal seizure (box) is seen. (**B**) Two detections (blue) and stimulations (arrow) are depicted and a seizure does not develop.

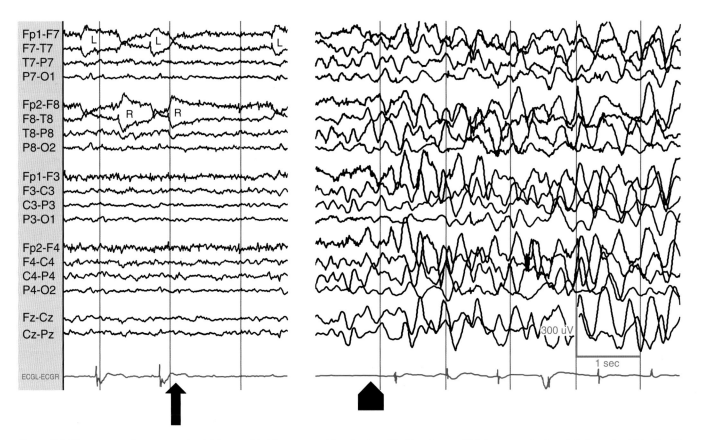

Figure 5-16 Pre-syncope due to asystole. A 14-year-old girl presents with episodes of feeling strange. EEG shows onset of asystole (arrow), which after 15 seconds (not shown) is followed by diffuse theta and delta slowing (arrowhead) consistent with global hypoperfusion. Asystole resolves at the moment of diffuse cerebral slowing and there is no LOC. Additionally, lateral eye movement artifact is seen with saccades to the right (R) and to the left (L).

153

Further reading

Alexopoulos, A., Jones, S., 2011. Focal motor seizures, epilepsia partialis continua, and supplementary sensorimotor seizures. In: Wyllie's Treatment of Epilepsy: Principles and Practice, 5th ed. Lippincott Williams & Wilkins, Philadelphia, PA.

Beaussart, M., 1972. Benign epilepsy of children with Rolandic (centro-temporal) paroxysmal foci. A clinical entity. Study of 221 cases. Epilepsia 13, 795–811.

Benbadis, S., 2011. Psychogenic nonepileptic attacks. In: Wyllie's Treatment of Epilepsy: Principles and Practice, 5th ed. Lippincott Williams & Wilkins, Philadelphia, PA.

Berg, A., Berkovic, S., Brodie, M., et al., 2010. Revised terminology and concepts for organization of seizures and epilepsies: Report of the ILAE Commission on Classification and Terminology, 2005–2009. Epilepsia 51 (4), 676–685.

Bodde, N.M., Brooks, J.L., Baker, G.A., et al., 2009. Psychogenic non-epileptic seizures – diagnostic issues: a critical review. Clin. Neurol. Neurosurg. 111 (1), 1–9.

Brenner, R.P., 2002. Is it status? Epilepsia 43 (Suppl. 3), 103–113.

Callaghan, N., Garrett, A., Googin, T., 1988. Withdrawal of anticonvulsant drugs in patients free of seizures for two years. N. Engl. J. Med. 318, 942–946.

Casino, G.D., 1993. Nonconvulsive status epilepticus in adults and children. Epilepsia 34, 781–784.

D'Argenzio, L., Cross, H., 2011. Hippocampal sclerosis and dual pathology. In: Wyllie's Treatment of Epilepsy: Principles and Practice, 5th ed. Lippincott Williams & Wilkins, Philadelphia, PA.

Delgado-Escueta, A.V., Enrile-Bacsal, F., 1984. Juvenile myoclonic epilepsy of Janz. Neurology 34, 285–294.

Devinsky, O., Cilio, M.R., Cross, H., et al., 2014. Cannabidiol: pharmacolog and potential therapeutic role in epilepsy and other neuropsychiatric disorders. Epilepsia 55 (6), 791–802.

Dubeau, F., 2011. Rasmussen encephalitis (chronic focal encephalitis). In: Wyllie's Treatment of Epilepsy: Principles and Practice, 5th ed. Lippincott Williams & Wilkins, Philadelphia, PA.

Engel, J., 2006. ILAE classification of epilepsy syndromes. Epilepsy Res. 70S, S5–S10.

Fisher, R.S., Boas, W.V.E., Blume, W., et al., 2005. Epileptic seizures and epilepsy: definitions proposed by the International League Against Epilepsy (ILAE) and the International Bureau for Epilepsy (IBE). Epilepsia 46, 470–472.

Gastaut, H., 1982. A new type of epilepsy: benign partial epilepsy of childhood with occipital spike-waves. Clin. EEG. 13, 13–22.

Hirsch, L., Gaspard, N., 2013. Status epilepticus. Continuum (N Y) 19 (3), 767–794.

Juul-Jensen, P., 1964. Frequency of seizure recurrence after discontinuance of anticonvulsant medication in patients with epileptic seizures. Epilepsia 5, 352–363.

Kellinghaus, C., LuDers, H., 2011. Classification of seizures. In: Wyllie's Treatment of Epilepsy: Principles and Practice, 5th ed. Lippincott Williams & Wilkins, Philadelphia, PA.

Lowenstein, D.H., Bleck, T., Macdonald, R.L., 1999. It's time to revise the definition of status epilepticus. Epilepsia 40 (1), 120–122.

Medical Research Council Antiepileptic Drug Withdrawal Study Group, 1991. Randomized study of antiepileptic drug withdrawal in patients in remission. Lancet 337, 1175–1180.

Mikata, M., Winchester, S., 2011. Continuous spike wave of slow sleep and Landau–Kleffner syndrome. In: Wyllie's Treatment of Epilepsy: Principles and Practice, 5th ed. Lippincott Williams & Wilkins, Philadelphia, PA.

Neubauer, B., Hahn, A., Tuxhorn, I., 2011. Progressive and infantile myoclonic epilepsies. In: Wyllie's Treatment of Epilepsy: Principles and Practice, 5th ed. Lippincott Williams & Wilkins, Philadelphia, PA.

Panayiotopoulos, C.P., 1989. Benign childhood epilepsy with occipital paroxysms: a 15-year prospective study. Ann. Neurol. 26, 51–56.

Porter, R.J., Penry, J.K., 1983. Petit mal status. Adv. Neurol. 34, 61–67.

Serviss, G.P., 1911. A trip of terror. In: A Columbus of space. Appleton, New York, NY, pp. 17–32.

Shafer, S.Q., Hauser, W.A., Annegers, J.F., et al., 1988. EEG and other early predictors of epilepsy remission: a community study. Epilepsia 29, 580–600.

Shinnar, S., Vining, E.P.G., Mellits, E.D., et al., 1985. Discontinuing antiepileptic medication in children with epilepsy after two years without seizures. N. Engl. J. Med. 313, 976–980.

Tatum, W., 2011. Atypical absence seizures, myoclonic, tonic, and atonic seizures. In: Wyllie's Treatment of Epilepsy: Principles and Practice, 5th ed. Lippincott Williams & Wilkins, Philadelphia, PA.

Tenney, J.R., Glauser, T.A., 2013. The current state of absence epilepsy: can we have your attention? Epilepsy Curr. 13 (3), 135–140.

Treiman, D.M., Meyers, P.D., Walton, N.Y., et al., 1998. Treatment of generalized convulsive status epilepticus: a randomized double-blind comparison of four intravenous regimens. N. Engl. J. Med. 339, 792–798.

Tuxhorn, I., 2011. Epileptic spasms. In: Wyllie's Treatment of Epilepsy: Principles and Practice, 5th ed. Lippincott Williams & Wilkins, Philadelphia, PA, p. 2011.

Wilson, J.V., Reynolds, E.H., 1990. Translation and analysis of a cuneiform text forming part of a Babylonian treatise on epilepsy. 1990. Med. Hist. 34, 185–198.

Winesett, P., Tatum, W., 2011. Encephalopathic generalized epilepsy and Lennox–Gastaut syndrome. In: Wyllie's Treatment of Epilepsy: Principles and Practice, 5th ed. Lippincott Williams & Wilkins, Philadelphia, PA.

Xiao, F., An, D., Deng, H., et al., 2014. Evaluation of levetiracetam and valproic acid as low-dose monotherapies for children with typical benign childhood epilepsy with centrotemporal spikes (BECTS). Seizure 23 (9), 756–761.

The EEG in other neurological and medical conditions and in status epilepticus 6

THE DEMENTIAS

There are many subtypes of dementias, and EEGs are nonspecific, often showing slowing of the PDR, loss of the usual anterior beta activity, and a gradual increase in diffuse slowing. Nevertheless, certain EEG features can help with our understanding of the problem. For example, focal slowing is most prominent in the anterior regions in frontotemporal dementia. In its early stages, Alzheimer's disease may display little or no EEG abnormality. As the disease progresses, first there is slowing of the PDR, which may eventually be lost entirely. Epileptiform discharges may appear later in the process and may be focal, generalized, or even periodic (Figure 6-1). Note that clinical seizures, generalized or focal, become more common as dementia progresses – particularly in its late stages.

Multi-infarct dementia (MID) is difficult to differentiate from other types of dementias on clinical grounds, as well as on EEG grounds. In MID the record is more likely to display asymmetric features. This no doubt results from multiple small strokes in the course of the illness.

Creutzfeldt–Jakob disease (CJD) has distinctive EEG and clinical characteristics. In the first place, the disease is rapidly progressive with cognitive decline and parallel EEG changes. The background rhythms become fragmented and are destroyed. Diffuse slowing appears and increases. Later, the distinctive periodic sharp wave discharges, often at 1 Hz, are recorded (Figure 6-2). At first, the discharges may be more irregular and even focal, only later becoming generalized and synchronous. Background activity decreases in amplitude. Eventually the EEG is dominated by the periodic discharges with no discernible background. Before death there is a decline in, and ultimate disappearance of, the discharges, leaving an essentially featureless record. A clinical note: the appearance of periodicity is commonly associated with myoclonus. Although the periodic sharp waves are associated with myoclonus, they are not usually time-locked with the myoclonus.

ISCHEMIC STROKE

Many patients presenting with acute ischemic stroke are relatively easy to diagnose on clinical grounds with respect to the history and physical examination. (Note to our readers: the neurological examination still retains its importance!) Others are less straightforward, and the clinician depends on an imaging study to aid in accurate diagnosis. In an acute

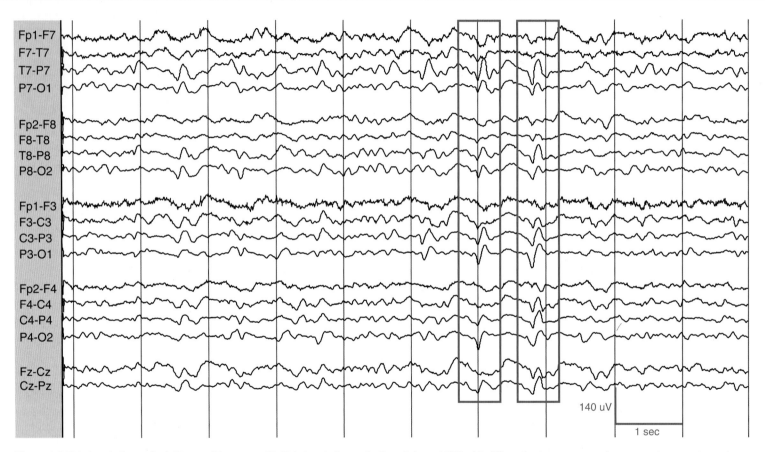

Figure 6-1 Alzheimer's dementia. A 90-year-old woman with Alzheimer's dementia. There is loss of PDR with diffuse slowing, most prominent over the posterior region. Generalized sharp waves are posteriorly predominant (boxes).

158

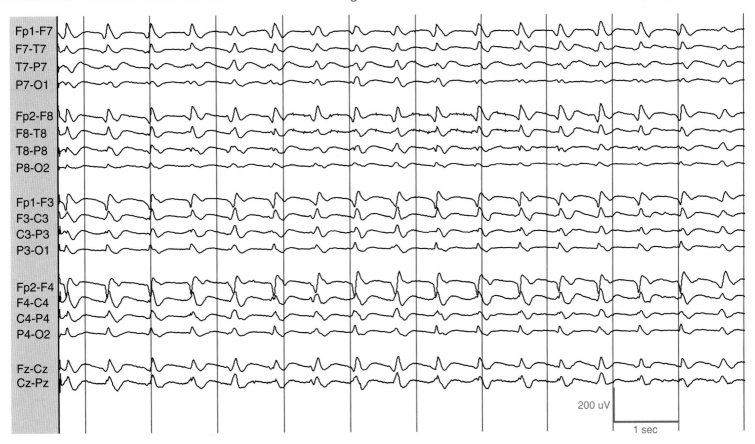

Figure 6-2 Creutzfeldt–Jakob disease (CJD). The EEG shows generalized periodic sharp waves at 1–2 Hz that are either biphasic or triphasic (GPDs) on a suppressed background in this 64-year-old woman with CJD.

cortical stroke, the CT of the brain may be normal while the EEG shows a focal decrease of amplitude from a reduction of cortical electrical production (Figure 6-3). Note that a similar voltage attenuation can be seen when there is an increase in fluid or blood between the cortex and the electrodes (e.g., subdural hematoma). These two conditions are hard to differentiate just from an EEG. Asymmetry of beta rhythms with reduction of amplitude is the earliest and most sensitive indicator of cortical dysfunction or a local cortical lesion. Then, polymorphic focal slow waves may appear in an area of reduced amplitude, suggesting that white matter under the cortex is involved as well. In some patients with acute infarction, epileptiform potentials (sharp waves and/or spikes) may be recorded. Further, the EEG sometimes reveals a pattern of lateralized periodic discharges (LPDs).

For example, the usual EEG picture in cases of middle cerebral artery occlusion reveals reduction of fast frequencies and an irregular or polymorphic delta focus in the involved hemisphere, maximal in frontal, temporal, and parietal regions. In addition, the PDR is usually disrupted. During sleep, depression of sleep spindles and vertex sharp waves on the side of the stroke may provide additional evidence of focal cerebral dysfunction.

When edema supervenes, the slowing may be more profound. Indeed, if the patient is lethargic, possibly due to midline intracranial shift, the opposite hemisphere will also demonstrate slowing and disorganization. Associated increased intracranial pressure or infarcts in the deep white matter may be accompanied by intermittent frontally predominant generalized rhythmic delta activity (GRDA).

Occipital strokes present a different picture. Slowing over the posterior temporal and occipital regions may be evident along with the ipsilateral reduction or destruction of the PDR (Figure 6-4). Note that photic stimulation may evoke an asymmetric driving response with depression over the involved side.

When the eyes open, the PDR attenuates in most normal controls. Unilateral failure of this attenuation can be caused by ipsilateral parietal and temporal lobe lesions. This can be an early and subtle sign of stroke or other lesion and is commonly known as Bancaud's phenomenon. Occlusion of the anterior cerebral artery usually results in frontal slowing, sometimes with frontal lateralized rhythmic delta activity (LRDA) or even frontally predominant GRDA. In such cases the occipital rhythms are preserved.

Many strokes are subcortical with sparing of the overlying cortex. Lacunar strokes involving the internal capsule or basal ganglia are common in patients with hypertension and are not always easy to differentiate clinically from those with cortical/subcortical involvement. Instead of demonstrating focal slowing, the record in these patients is usually normal. Alternatively, it may contain a mild diffuse abnormality without lateralizing features.

Patients with clinically suspected transient ischemic attacks are often referred for an EEG. In these cases the record is usually normal or nonfocal if obtained after resolution of the neurological findings. In some cases, however, intermittent focal slowing may be evident, suggesting that residual cerebral dysfunction is indeed present despite a normal neurological examination. If the EEG is obtained while the patient is symptomatic, appropriate focal slowing may be evident.

HEMORRHAGIC STROKE

Hemorrhagic strokes present a highly variable EEG picture depending on the site of involvement, extent of the pathology, and the patient's state of awareness. A relatively small hemorrhage in the centrum semiovale likely results in a minor degree of lateralized slowing. On the other hand, basal ganglia hemorrhages with obtundation can demonstrate marked disruption of electrocortical activity with bilateral delta activity.

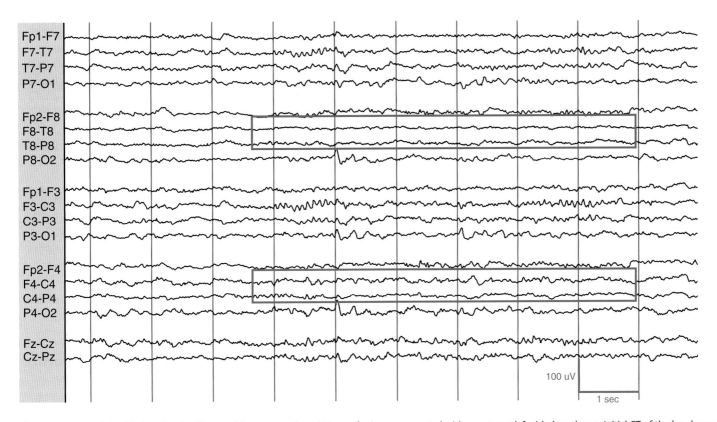

Figure 6-3 Acute right-sided stroke. An 83-year-old woman with no history of seizures presented with new-onset left-sided weakness. Initial CT of the head was negative for acute findings. EEG during sleep shows attenuation of fast frequencies and loss of sleep spindles over the right hemisphere (boxes), concerning for an acute stroke. (Intervening fluid collection such as subdural hematoma can have similar findings, but this was ruled out by the CT head.) Repeat head CT the following day confirmed an acute right middle cerebral artery ischemic stroke.

161

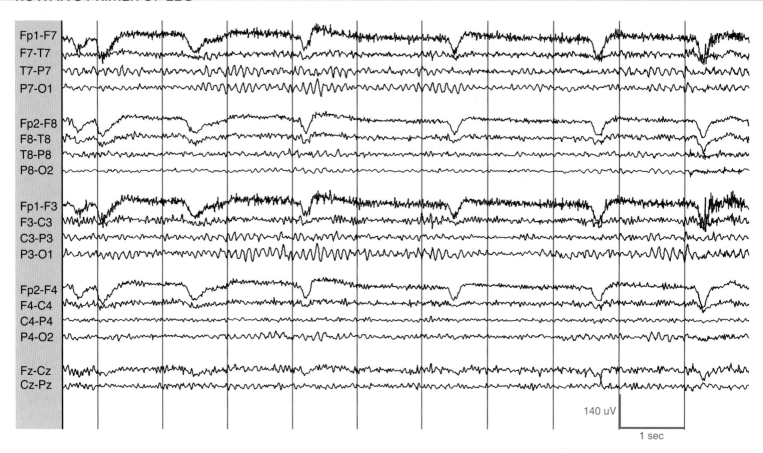

Figure 6-4 Chronic right occipital stroke. An 84-year-old woman with a chronic right occipital stroke. There is an asymmetry of the PDR, with the left PDR being more than twice the amplitude of the right PDR. Higher amplitude on the right is commonly seen in normal subjects, and this is more than the allowable amplitude asymmetry.

162

Lateralization to the involved side may be seen, although in the face of depressed consciousness asymmetry may not be evident. GRDA is common in such cases.

SUBDURAL HEMATOMA

The classic EEG finding in subdural hematoma (SDH) is depression of cerebral activity over the involved hemisphere. This so-called insulation defect consists of reduced amplitude as compared with the opposite hemisphere. In addition, the PDR may be disrupted or even absent. If the collection is large, associated slowing may be evident. It should be emphasized that there is considerable variability in the EEG, and the classic finding of background depression is not always seen. If the SDH is small there may be no obvious EEG findings.

We also find unilateral depression of cerebral activity in subdural hygromas and atrophic processes secondary to congenital brain damage. In addition, porencephaly leads to striking depression of the background that may present an essentially isopotential (flat) picture.

METABOLIC DISORDERS

Clinically metabolic disorders can result in a mildly altered mental status, personality changes, or even coma. The hallmark of a metabolic encephalopathy is diffuse slowing. In addition, the PDR is invariably disrupted and slowed or is absent. The slowing may be mild or profound, depending on the extent of the encephalopathy and the level of consciousness. The slowing is usually symmetric unless there is an underlying focal cerebral lesion unrelated to the metabolic disorder. In such cases one may see focal and diffuse slowing. While recording, the technologist should attempt to arouse the patient. This may result in an increase in the background frequency, which is a demonstration of EEG reactivity.

In addition to diffuse slowing, frontally predominant GRDA may be recorded. Note that frontally predominant GRDA is a non-specific finding and may also be seen in intoxications, increased intracranial pressure, and deep structural lesions.

An important feature of metabolic encephalopathies is triphasic waves, which can become periodic (GPDs with triphasic morphology) (Figure 6-5). Classically, the initial deflection of this triphasic wave is negative (upgoing) and brief, the second deflection is positive (downgoing) and a bit longer in duration, and the third deflection is negative (upgoing) and the slowest. In addition, the classic metabolic triphasic wave demonstrates an anterior-posterior delay, that is, the frontal component leads the posterior component by 100 ms or so. The underlying neurophysiological reason for the front-to-back delay is not understood. GPDs with triphasic morphology are classically seen in hepatic encephalopathy but can be seen with uremia, sepsis, and electrolyte disturbances. However, biphasic generalized sharp waves, focal and multifocal epileptiform potentials, and focal and generalized seizures can be seen in toxic metabolic states.

It can be quite difficult on visual inspection to delineate between GPDs secondary to a toxic metabolic cause and GPDs, which may in fact represent non-convulsive status epilepticus (NCSE). The two conditions may have a strikingly similar EEG appearance, though there is usually no anterior-posterior delay in NCSE. GPDs that are faster in frequency (>3 Hz) or have evolution meet the criteria for electrographic seizures.

COMA

In coma, the EEG can show a wide variety of patterns including, *but not limited to*, alpha coma, burst-suppression, or even NCSE. The

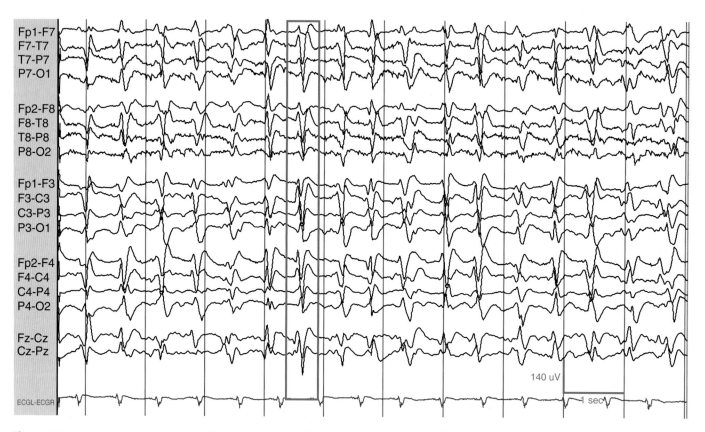

Figure 6-5 Generalized periodic discharges (GPDs) with a mostly triphasic morphology. A 66-year-old woman with a history of breast cancer presented with altered mental status. EEG shows continuous generalized periodic sharp waves of mostly triphasic morphology, occurring at 2 Hz. An example of a triphasic wave with an anterior to posterior lag is seen in the box.

clinical examination can be identical for all of these patterns, and the approach to the patient and prognosis varies depending on the EEG findings and etiology of the coma.

NON-REACTIVE EEG

The EEG is said to be reactive when there is a change in cerebral rhythm to stimulation, which includes change in amplitude or frequency. Eye blink artifacts or muscle artifacts do not count. To aid in correct interpretation of the EEG, it is important for the EEG technician to stimulate comatose patients (noxious stimulation/passive eye opening) and note the time of stimulation on EEG.

Alpha coma

This is a distinct EEG constellation, usually resulting from widespread cerebral damage (as from anoxia). In this case, the rhythmic alpha characteristically appears most prominently in the frontal derivations but may be diffusely represented. There is no response to external stimuli or passive opening of the eyes. Sleep wake cycles are absent. These findings usually imply a poor prognosis despite the lack of any diffuse slowing. If the alpha is more dominant posteriorly (as is seen in the normal population) and attenuates with alerting stimuli, the possibility of a patient in a locked-in state should be entertained.

Theta or delta coma

If the background shows predominantly delta or theta activity, the coma can be termed a delta/theta coma. This pattern is seen in a wide variety of etiologies, and the prognosis largely depends on the etiology.

Spindle coma

In spindle coma, the EEG includes prominent spindle-like activity, similar to that seen in stage 2 sleep. It is typically seen with high mesencephalic lesions and portends a better outcome than alpha coma.

Beta coma

Beta coma is characterized by high-amplitude beta activity, sometimes frontally predominant. Beta coma is often the result of intoxication with barbiturates or benzodiazepines, and it generally portends a favorable outcome.

BURST-SUPPRESSION

The term burst-suppression refers to a cycling of marked depression of cerebral activity and bursts of cerebral activity of variable amplitude, duration, and waveform (Figure 6-6). The bursts may be composed of multiphasic delta components, admixtures of various frequencies, or epileptiform activity such as spikes or sharp waves, often with admixed slow components. According to the ACNS terminology, more than 50% of the record consists of suppression, alternating with bursts lasting 0.5–30 seconds. The prototype of this phenomenon is found in patients receiving general anesthesia. It is thought that burst-suppression results from suppression of cortical activity via GABA-ergic mechanisms with breakthrough EEG activity due to intact glutaminergic transmission. Under progressively deepening anesthesia there are sequential EEG changes from normal sleep patterns, to diffuse delta waves, then burst-suppression, and finally isopotentiality. The burst-suppression pattern is medically induced, often with anesthetics, in patients with refractory status epilepticus or other conditions in which it is desirable to lower metabolic demand of the brain.

Burst-suppression also occurs in patients with cardiopulmonary arrest who suffer from cerebral anoxia. In this case, the prognosis is usually poor, and often generalized or lateralized epileptiform discharges are seen within the bursts, which can have correlation with clinical myoclonus. Burst-suppression may also be encountered in neonates, usually those with severe cerebral damage or certain rare syndromes. The prognosis in such cases is usually poor.

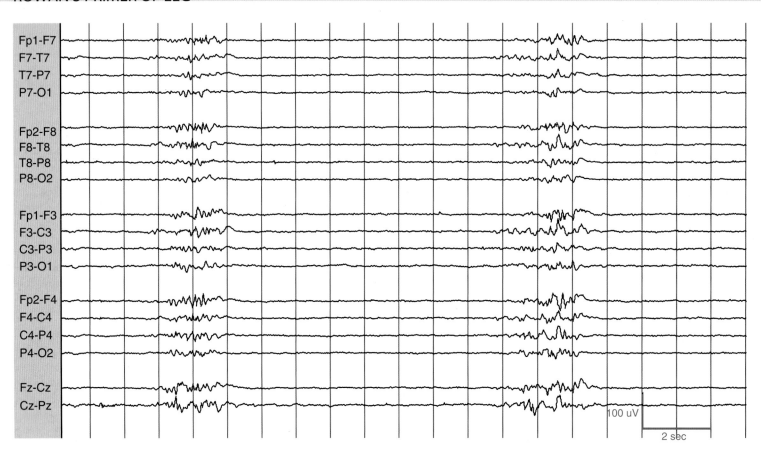

Figure 6-6 Burst suppression pattern. 74-year-old woman in a sedated coma for the treatment of NCSE in the medical intensive care unit. The bursts consist of a mixture of theta and delta frequencies lasting 1–2 seconds, which alternates with periods of suppression lasting for 6–12 seconds.

STATUS EPILEPTICUS

"If the possessing demon possesses him many times during the middle watch of the night, and at the time of his possession his hands and feet are cold, he is much darkened, keeps opening and shutting his mouth … It may go on for some time, but he will die."–From a tablet written in Babylon in 600–700 BC.

Status epilepticus, ongoing intermittent or continuous uncontrolled seizures, has long been recognized to pose severe danger to the individual in its grips. Several millennia after this quote was written on a cuneiform tablet in Babylon, status epilepticus still causes significant mortality and morbidity. The question becomes: At what point does a seizure become status? Previously, the standard definition was ongoing clinical seizure activity lasting longer than 30 minutes or multiple discrete seizures without return to baseline functioning. However, the average length of a GTCC is less than 2 minutes and the exact moment of irreversible neuronal injury is not known, *likely varying* between individuals. A more practical definition is ongoing seizure activity for greater than 5 minutes or multiple discrete seizures without returning to a baseline mental status. This definition invites more aggressive treatment, and early treatment has been shown to be more effective in both animal models and humans.

Status epilepticus is an umbrella term for a wide range of clinical conditions with widely varying prognoses. Status epilepticus can be convulsive with overt clinical manifestations (such as GTCC, tonic or clonic seizures, myoclonic seizures, hemiconvulsive seizures) or have very subtle (such as minor facial twitching or nystagmoid jerking of the eyes) or no clinical manifestations (NCSE). Generalized tonic clonic status epilepticus is life threatening and requires swift and aggressive management with intubation and an IV anesthetic. More subtle status epilepticus, as in EPC, can occur in a perfectly alert and conversant individual and requires trials of various AEDs, often with the aim of avoiding intubation. In fact, essentially every seizure type (tonic–clonic, tonic, clonic, myoclonic, absence or focal) can become status epilepticus. The diagnosis can be elusive as people in focal status or even absence status may present with bizarre behavior and altered mentation. In addition, patients with lethargy, obtundation, or coma may well be having non-convulsive status epilepticus (NCSE). NCSE can occur after convulsive status epilepticus or without any prior clinical seizures. Any individual who has had clinical seizures and is not back to baseline should be urgently connected to VEEG as the distinction between a post-ictal state and ongoing seizure activity cannot be made clinically.

Status epilepticus commonly occurs in critically ill patients. NCSE is especially common in critically ill patients, and in fact, most seizures (about 75% on average in the literature) that occur in these patients are non-convulsive and cannot be identified without an EEG. In any patient who is critically ill with a depressed level of consciousness, with or without known neurological problems, NCSE should be on the differential. It is particularly important as NCSE is a potentially treatable cause of obtundation and coma.

Unequivocal electrographic seizures are defined as (1) generalized or focal spike-wave discharges at 3 Hz or faster (Figure 6-7); and (2) clearly evolving discharges of any type that reach a frequency of more than 4Hz, whether generalized or focal (Figure 6-8A).

An EEG pattern is said to evolve if there are at least two unequivocal sequential changes in frequency, morphology, or location. When the EEG pattern does not meet the above criteria, it does not mean that it is not a seizure; it may or may not be. We know that at least 6 cm^2 of cortex needs to be involved to see seizures on surface electrodes. Intracranial EEG recordings, with electrodes on the surface of the brain or within the brain (depth electrodes), can show focal seizures that are not seen on surface extracranial electrodes.

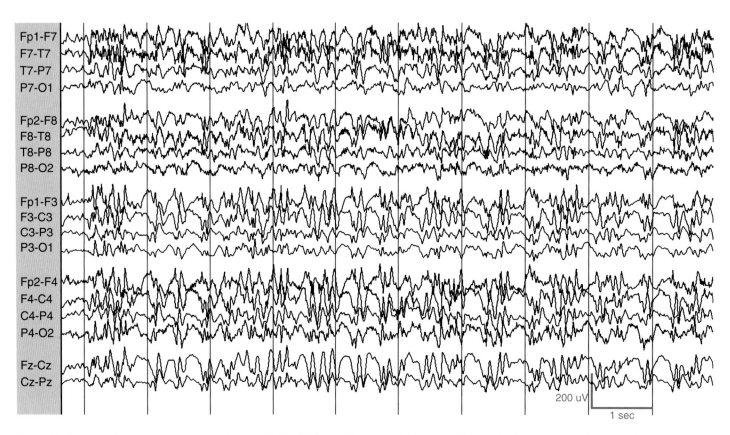

Figure 6-7 Generalized non-convulsive status epilepticus (NCSE). A 56-year-old woman with a history of generalized epilepsy was admitted with altered mental status and no verbal output. EEG revealed nearly continuous generalized spike/polyspike/sharp and wave discharges at medium to high amplitude, fluctuating in frequencies up to 7 Hz, meeting the criteria for non-convulsive status epilepticus.

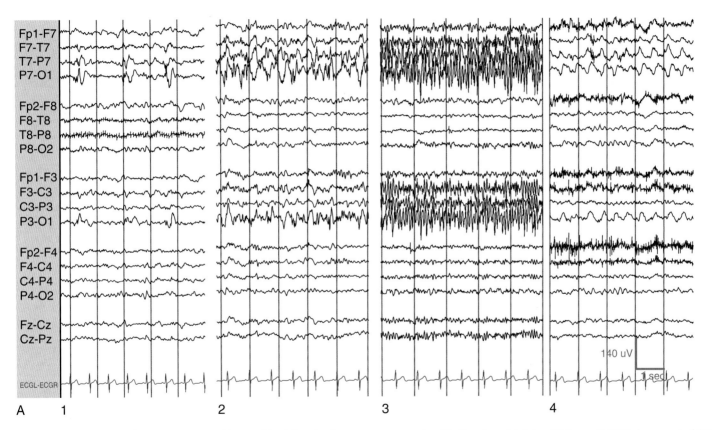

Figure 6-8 Focal status epilepticus. A 62-year-old man with a left parietal astrocytoma presents with altered mental status. (**A**) Sequential EEG shows an evolving focal seizure. The seizure starts with left posterior periodic sharp waves and spikes (LPDs) (1), which become faster in frequency (2) with spread to other regions in the left hemisphere (3). Postictally, there is rhythmic delta activity over the left posterior region (LRDA) (4).

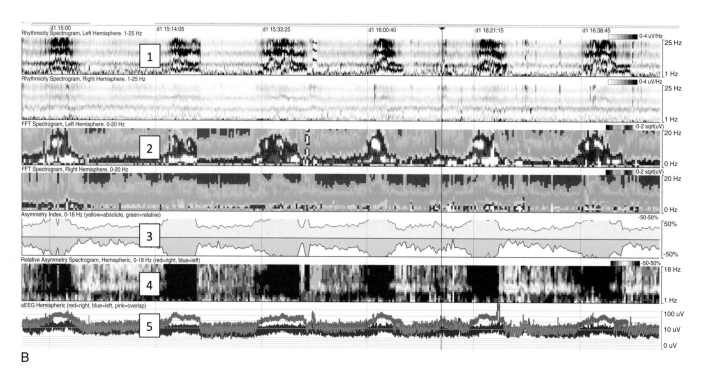

Figure 6-8, cont'd (**B**) Quantitative EEG (QEEG) showing 2 hours of recording. (1) The rhythmicity spectrogram picks up increased rhythmicity in the record. Six left hemisphere (top band) seizures are clearly evident. (2) Fast Fourier transform (FFT) spectrogram uses color to display the power in the EEG at certain frequencies. Frequencies in the bandwidth from 0–20 Hz are represented in the vertical axis. During each seizure, there is increased power at both lower and higher frequencies on the left. White represents the highest power. (3) Asymmetry index. During each seizure for this patient, the hemispheres become increasingly asymmetric from one another. (4) Relative asymmetry spectrogram. This band shows that even between seizures, there is more power on the left (left = blue; right = red). During each seizure, the blue is darker, indicating an even greater difference between the hemispheres, with more power on the left. (5) Average EEG looking at amplitude (left = blue, right=red). When the color is fuchsia, the hemispheres are roughly equivalent in amplitude. During the seizures, the left hemisphere is clearly higher in amplitude.

As discussed in Chapter 4, certain electrographic features are considered more likely to be ictal. For example, when PDs are associated with superimposed fast frequency (+F), this pattern is considered more likely to be ictal than a pattern with PDs without +F. When the pattern is unclear (fair warning: the patterns are often not clear!) and the patient is obtunded, one may try administering a fast-acting AED and observe for clinical and electrographic improvements. If improvement occurs (particularly clinical improvement), the pattern should be considered NCSE. For EEG patterns in the gray zone, the term ictal–interictal continuum is sometimes used. In critically ill patients, many findings can be missed from routine EEGs and it is recommended to do long-term EEG monitoring, especially if rhythmic or periodic patterns are present, because these are associated with increased risk of seizures.

For critically ill patients who are on long-term EEG monitoring, many patterns can be identified by using programs that quantify and compress EEG data (e.g., quantitative EEG; QEEG). Typically, several hours of EEG data are compressed to fit on the screen. Various compressed EEG trends can allow for clear portrayal of status epilepticus, early stroke, deepening sedation, etc. For example, once a given compressed pattern (this can be highly recognizable) is confirmed to represent a seizure by an experienced epileptologist reviewing the raw EEG data, the staff in an ICU can be instructed to titrate medication until that seizure fingerprint remits (Figure 6-8B).

Status epilepticus can occur in individuals who are medically ill, neurologically ill (brain tumor, stroke), and in patients with known epilepsy. In patients with epilepsy, status epilepticus typically happens because of the *refractory nature of the epilepsy* or because of medication non-compliance. In addition, epilepsy can present with status epilepticus. Rarely, individuals will present with new-onset refractory status epilepticus (NORSE) whose etiology is unclear (Figure 6-9). Status epilepticus in individuals who do not have known epilepsy should be evaluated for an underlying disorder like meningitis, encephalitis, sepsis, brain trauma, metabolic derangements or stroke. In those cases, treatment of the status epilepticus is two pronged: the individual is managed with AEDs (including anesthetic infusions if necessary) and aggressive treatment of the underlying process. For example, in an individual who presents in status with auto-immune limbic encephalitis, appropriate treatment includes AEDs and high-dose steroids. Treatment of status epilepticus is outlined in Appendix 2.

BRAIN DEATH

Brain death is essentially a clinical diagnosis. Under certain circumstances, an EEG might be ordered to confirm the diagnosis. Electrocerebral inactivity (ECI) is defined as the absence of any waves of cerebral origin. The record should not have activity that exceeds 2 μV, unless that activity is clear environmental artifact (e.g., an IV drip or cardiac artifact). Low-frequency filters should be set between 0.5 Hz and 1.5 Hz, and the high-frequency filter should be set at 70 Hz. For a brain death examination, the interelectrode impedance should be between 1000 and 10,000 Ohms. The EEG should be reviewed at a sensitivity of 2 μV/mm for at least 30 minutes, and a double-distance bipolar montage should be available to maximize the chances of detecting cerebral activity. In order to call this ECI consistent with brain death, reversible disturbances must be excluded (toxic–metabolic perturbations, hypothermia, or sedating medication).

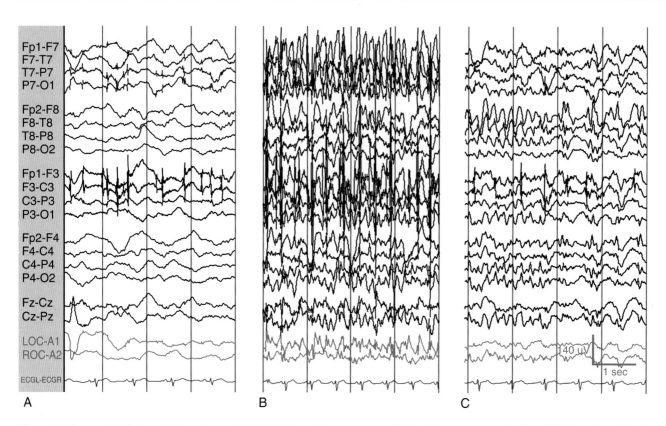

Figure 6-9 New-onset refractory status epilepticus (NORSE). 31-year-old man presented with refractory status epilepticus. (**A**) Shows the artifact from ongoing left face twitching. There is no electrographic right-sided seizure evident. (**B**) Hours later, he developed left facial twitching, which was more vigorous, and right hemisphere rhythmic activity can be discerned. (**C**) Ongoing right-sided electrographic seizure activity with a few facial twitches. Phenytoin, levetiracetam, midazolam, and ketamine failed to control his seizure activity, and he was placed in a pentobarbital coma.

Further reading

Beniczky, S., Hirsch, L.J., Kaplan, P.W., et al., 2013. Unified EEG terminology and criteria for nonconvulsive status epilepticus. Epilepsia 54 (Suppl. 6), 28–29.

Bickford, R.G., Butt, H.R., 1955. Hepatic coma: the electroencephalographic pattern. J. Clin. Invest. 34 (6), 790–799.

Brenner, R.P., 1985. The electroencephalogram in altered states of consciousness. Neurol. Clin. Invest. 3 (3), 615–631.

Britt, C.W., Jr., 1981. Nontraumatic "spindle coma": clinical, EEG, and prognostic features. Neurology 31 (4), 393–397.

Burger, L.J., Rowan, A.J., Goldensohn, E.S., 1972. Creutzfeldt–Jakob disease. An electroencephalographic study. Arch. Neurol. 26 (5), 428–433.

Celesia, G.G., 1973. Pathophysiology of periodic EEG complexes in subacute sclerosing panencehalitis (SSPE). Electroencephalogr. Clin. Neurophysiol. 35 (3), 293–300.

Chiofalo, N., Fuentes, A., Galvez, S., 1980. Serial EEG findings in 27 cases of Creutzfeldt–Jakob disease. Arch. Neurol. 37 (3), 143–145.

Claassen, J., Hirsch, L.J., Kreiter, K.T., et al., 2004. Quantitative continuous EEG for detecting delayed cerebral ischemia in patients with poor-grade subarachnoid hemorrhage. Clin. Neurophysiol. 115 (12), 2699–2710.

Claassen, J., Jette, N., Chum, F., et al., 2007. Electrographic seizures and periodic discharges after intracerebral hemorrhage. Neurology 69 (13), 1356–1365.

Claassen, J., Mayer, S.A., Kowalski, R.G., et al., 2004. Detection of electrographic seizures with continuous EEG monitoring in critically ill patients. Neurology 62 (10), 1743–1748.

DeLorenzo, R.J., Waterhouse, E.J., Towne, A.R., et al., 1998. Persistent nonconvulsive status epilepticus after the control of convulsive status epilepticus. Epilepsia 39 (8), 833–840.

Hirsch, L.J., Gaspard, N., 2013. Status epilepticus. Continuum (N Y) 19 (3 Epilepsy), 767–794.

Husain, A.M., 2006. Electroencephalographic assessment of coma. J. Clin. Neurophysiol. 23 (3), 208–220.

Kaplan, P.W., Genoud, D., Ho, T.W., et al., 1999. Etiology, neurologic correlations, and prognosis in alpha coma. Clin. Neurophysiol. 110 (2), 205–213.

Lai, C.W., Gragasin, M.E., 1988. Electroencephalography in herpes simplex encephalitis. J. Clin. Neurophysiol. 5 (1), 87–103.

Levy, S.R., Chiappa, K.H., Burke, C.J., et al., 1986. Early evolution and incidence of electroencephalographic abnormalities in Creutzfeldt–Jakob disease. J. Clin. Neurophysiol. 3 (1), 1–21.

Lowenstein, D.H., Aminoff, M.J., 1992. Clinical and EEG features of status epilepticus in comatose patients. Neurology 42 (1), 100–104.

Mayer, S.A., Claassen, J., Lokin, J., et al., 2002. Refractory status epilepticus: frequency, risk factors, and impact on outcome. Arch. Neurol. 59 (2), 205–210.

Mecarelli, O., Pro, S., Randi, F., et al., 2011. EEG patterns and epileptic seizures in acute phase stroke. Cerebrovasc. Dis. 31 (2), 191–198.

Petty, G.W., Labar, D.R., Fisch, B.J., et al., 1995. Electroencephalography in lacunar infarction. J. Neurol. Sci. 134 (1–2), 47–50.

Roberts, M.A., McGeorge, A.P., Caird, F.I., 1978. Electroencephalography and computerised tomography in vascular and non-vascular dementia in old age. J. Neurol. Neurosurg. Psychiatry. 41 (10), 903–906.

Stewart, C.P., Otsubo, H., Ochi, A., et al., 2010. Seizure identification in the ICU using quantitative EEG displays. Neurology 75 (17), 1501–1508.

Tay, S.K., Hirsch, L.J., Leary, L., et al., 2006. Nonconvulsive status epilepticus in children: clinical and EEG characteristics. Epilepsia 47 (9), 1504–1509.

Towne, A.R., Waterhouse, E.J., Boggs, J.G., et al., 2000. Prevalence of nonconvulsive status epilepticus in comatose patients. Neurology 54 (2), 340–345.

Treiman, D.M., Meyers, P.D., Walton, N.Y., et al., 1996. Treatment of generalized convulsive status epilepticus: A multicenter comparison of four drug regimens. Neurology 46 (2), 150–153.

Treiman, D.M., Walton, N.Y., Kendrick, C., 1990. A progressive sequence of electroencephalographic changes during generalized convulsive status epilepticus. Epilepsy Res. 5 (1), 49–60.

Walsh, J.M., Brenner, R.P., 1987. Periodic lateralized epileptiform discharges – long-term outcome in adults. Epilepsia 28 (5), 533–536.

Young, G.B., Blume, W.T., Campbell, V.M., et al., 1994. Alpha, theta and alpha-theta coma: a clinical outcome study utilizing serial recordings. Electroencephalogr. Clin. Neurophysiol. 91 (2), 93–99.

The EEG: Tips on indications, reading, and reporting

7

INDICATIONS

ROUTINE EEG

- Initial assessment for patients with possible epilepsy or after a seizure. If normal, depending on the level of suspicion, a repeat routine EEG, a sleep-deprived study, or a long-term EEG may be indicated.
- Follow-up assessment after the introduction of AEDs.
- Follow-up assessment after the cessation of AEDs.

INPATIENT VEEG MONITORING

- Characterization of seizures in a person with known epilepsy who is undergoing a pre-surgical evaluation.
- Determination of seizure frequency when undetected seizures are suspected. For example, if a patient with known epilepsy is having worsened memory problems, there may be subclinical seizures worsening cognition.
- Distinguishing between epileptic, psychogenic non-epileptic attacks (PNEA), and other seizure mimics.

- Changing medications in a controlled and safe environment for those with refractory epilepsy.
- Management of ongoing seizures or status epilepticus.
- Ongoing monitoring in patients with lethargy, obtundation, and coma to ascertain if the altered level of consciousness is caused by ongoing seizures.

If seizure characterization is desired, various provocation techniques are carried out during the study, including hyperventilation, photic stimulation, and sleep deprivation.

AMBULATORY EEG (AEEG) MONITORING

This long-term monitoring technique has the attraction of sending the patient home with a small, portable EEG amplifier with or without a camera. Typically, the patient carries out normal activities and keeps a diary of any events that occur. Recording may be carried out for days. Family members or friends can aid in the note keeping as the patient may be unaware of events. Indications are more constricted than the indications for in-patient VEEG, as it is not appropriate to stop medications to capture seizures at home or (obviously) to manage status epilepticus at home.

HOW TO LOOK AT THE RECORD

The beginner electroencephalographer is faced with an endless array of wiggly lines, and the meaning behind those lines can be elusive. The task of discerning clinically relevant information seems, at first, impossible. Like learning to read musical notes or learning to read in a foreign language, the secret to success is practice and exposure. In addition, the electroencephalographer should develop an armature, or systematic underlying structure, on which the information in each EEG can be reported. This report provides useful information to the clinician with the goal of ultimately improving the quality of life of our patients.

In order to interpret the record properly, one must have clearly in mind the elements of a normal EEG. This establishes a template, against which all deviations are to be compared. It is useful to analyze carefully the first few interpretable epochs with the intention of creating a basic scaffold in which further details will be added later. One may begin to ascertain the background including systematic thought to the continuity, symmetry, organization, and reactivity of the record. Is there a reactive PDR? If there is no PDR, is the record reactive to stimulation? Technicians should give nailbed pressure and passively open and close the eyes in any patient who does not fully alert with voice or a gentle shake. Abnormalities may be glaring as in a burst suppression pattern. Or one may appreciate a hint of focality, a hint of paroxysmal activity, or a possible asymmetry of background activity. If the patient is awake at the onset of the EEG, it is good to repeat this careful analysis in the first epoch of sleep. The symmetry and presence of sleep transients (K-complexes, positive occipital sharp transients of sleep (POSTs), sleep spindles, vertex waves) should be noted, as well as the presence of sleep stages. Slow wave sleep (SWS) is not often seen in a routine EEG or in hospitalized patients. Stage II sleep is a particularly fruitful time for the appearance of epileptiform discharges, if present.

After the first few minutes of the EEG are scrutinized, the experienced electroencephalographer will often begin to speed through pages at a rapid rate. With wiggly lines racing by, the electroencephalographer is looking with a relaxed and alert gaze at the whole screen, perhaps looking softly from the left-sided electrodes to the right-sided electrodes. This is somewhat akin to what we feel when we drive a car; we are alert, we are looking ahead and we are ready to respond to anything unusual. When something does stand out from the background, the electroencephalographer will pause and focus. Perhaps the element that stood out from the background looks like a possible sharp wave. The wave should be scrutinized in different montages. First, the longitudinal bipolar montage, is there a phase reversal? If so, at what electrode(s)? Is there an aftergoing slow wave? Once this has been established, the wave should be examined in a referential montage with the hypothesis that the electrode with the phase reversal will have the highest amplitude in a reference montage (see Chapter 1). If the abnormality appears maximally either in the occipital or frontopolar electrodes, a circumferential montage should be used, as phase reversals will not be apparent on the longitudinal bipolar montage (because of the end of chain effect). Many things will catch the novice's eye (e.g., muscle artifacts and wicket spikes). Before an element is called epileptiform, it must stand up to scrutiny. If there are abundant epileptiform potentials on one side, it is often useful to re-read the record with focus and attention on the quieter hemisphere to make sure that sharp waves and spikes are not missed.

The electroencephalographer will stop for a seizure. In this case, the video is examined and then the EEG is examined in a very detailed manner. We seek to identify the exact electrographic onset, so it is necessary to backtrack from the obvious onset to see if there is perhaps a more subtle onset that was missed. The clinical description should include detailed notes, as semiology can help clinicians lateralize and even localize seizures.

If there is a flurry of movement artifact, the electroencephalographer should pause and look at the video (if present). EEGs are often ordered for an evaluation of an unusual movement, and any strange movements should be commented on in the report.

The EEG may be annotated with notes of clinical events reported by the patient, a family member, or the nursing staff. These events should be analyzed in detail. As mentioned in Chapter 5, the diagnosis often depends on the video as an event without EEG change can either be a surface negative seizure or a seizure mimic like PNEA. The semiology of the event can in most cases clarify the diagnosis. For all events, the EKG strip should be reviewed and any EKG correlates should be reported on.

ELEMENTS OF THE REPORT

Guidelines provided by the ACNS should be followed so that the nomenclature used in the EEG report is standardized (Table 4-1). After all, what one neurologist means by "frequent" may be different from what the next neurologist means by "frequent." Table 7-1 outlines a standard order for an EEG report.

Table 7-1 The EEG report	
TYPE OF RECORDING	The software, the number of electrodes used, the type of EEG (routine, sleep deprived, in-patient, long-term, intracranial etc), and the presence or absence of video should be noted. Any spike or event detection programs used should be noted. If the recording is intracranial, the electrode array should be described and a diagram should be attached at the end of the report.
CLINICAL INFORMATION	The patient's name, date of birth, medical record number, location, and total recording time should appear at the top of the report. In addition, the reason for the EEG request and any medications that affect the central nervous system are reported in this section.
FACTUAL REPORT	If the study is a multi-day study, this section of the report should be repeated for each day. Medication changes should be noted for each day.
Background	
Organization	In adults, the normal waking record contains a PDR (note the frequency in Hz), of maximum amplitude in the posterior quadrants. Beta activity is present frontocentrally, in greater or lesser amounts – this is the normal A-P gradient. Note presence or absence of the A-P gradient. If present, drowsiness and sleep are described. Sleep stages and transients are described. Features of organization of neonates and children are age specific (Chapter 3).
Symmetry/frequency	A description of the predominant frequencies is recorded. A comparison of frequency and amplitude is made between the left and right sides. Slowing, if present, is described in terms of location (generalized/focal), frequency, morphology (polymorphic/monomorphic), and quantity. RDA is placed in the section with epileptiform abnormalities as it can be a marker of cortical hyperexcitability. Breach artifacts (higher amplitude with increased frequency due to skull defects) are noted. Focal and generalized attenuation is noted.

Continued

Table 7-1 continued

Reactivity	In healthy patients this is typically easy to identify – when the eyes are closed in a relaxed awake state the PDR emerges. In comatose patients it is not as easy to determine and one must rely on the technician. The technician typically opens and closes a patient's eyes. In catatonic patients who do not seem to react, passive eye opening and closure will bring out a PDR. In comatose patients the technician should also administer noxious stimulation. Reactivity refers to a change in the brain waves, not in the appearance of eye blinks or muscle artifact. If only SIRPIDs are present, it should be reported as: reactive, SIRPIDS only.
Continuity	Specify if the background is continuous, nearly continuous, discontinuous, or in a burst-suppression pattern. Duration of bursts and interburst intervals are noted. Morphology of bursts is described.
Interictal epileptiform discharges, rhythmic or periodic patterns	List spikes, sharp waves, PDs, and RDA (both generalized and lateralized) in this section. Relative prevalence, frequency, morphology, location, duration, and presence in various states (sleep/wake/drowsiness) should be noted. Specify SIRPIDs, if present, and type of stimuli. *Example:* *1. Rare frontally predominant generalized spike and wave discharges at 3 Hz of very brief duration, present in sleep.* *2. Abundant right parietal (P4) spikes, predominantly in wakefulness.*
Activation procedures	Responses to photic stimulation and hyperventilation are described here.
Events/seizures	The time and duration of the event, clinical description, and EEG findings appear under this heading. In addition, if someone is in subclinical status, a brief picture of the overall neurological state is placed here (e.g., *"The patient was lethargic on this day, rousable with noxious but unable to follow commands"*). For discreet events, give specific times for the clinical and EEG progression. A detailed clinical description can aid in the diagnosis. For example, this clinical description is consistent with seizure, specifically epilepsia partialis continua (EPC), even though there is no electrographic correlate: *Continuous 1 Hz right hand clonic movements with supination are present. These persist in sleep and are not suppressible during examination.*
IMPRESSION	List in summary the essential findings. Findings should be listed in the same order as they appear in the body of the report. *Example: This is an abnormal EEG demonstrating*: *1. Frequent left polymorphic fontotemporal slowing.* *2. Abundant left anterior temporal spikes (T7) in wakefulness and sleep.* *3. A single brief seizure with unresponsiveness of left anterior temporal origin.*
CLINICAL CORRELATION	This final section is perhaps the most important aspect of the report. If the findings support a diagnosis of left temporal lobe epilepsy, say it here. If the findings are consistent with a metabolic disorder, or a structural lesion, then so indicate. If the findings are non-specific, then list a succinct differential. In this section of the report, slowing, either focal or generalized, is often referred to as cerebral dysfunction, whereas spikes, sharp waves, PDs, and LRDA are referred to as epileptiform potentials, cortical hyperexcitability, or cortical irritability.

RDA, rhythmic delta activity; PDR, posterior dominant rhythm; SIRPID, stimulation induced rhythmic, periodic, or ictal discharges; PD, periodic discharges; LRDA, lateralized rhythmic delta activity; A-P gradient, anterior to posterior gradient.

Further reading

American Clinical Neurophysiology Society Guidelines. <www.acns.org>.

American EEG Society Guidelines in Electroencephalography, Evoked Potentials and Polysomnography, 1994. Guideline Eight: Guidelines for writing EEG reports. J. Clin. Neurophysiol. 11, 37–39.

Kellaway, P., 1979. An orderly approach to visual analysis: parameters of the normal EEG in adults and children. In: Klass, D.W., Daly, D.D. (Eds.), Current Practice of Clinical Electroencephalography. Raven Press, New York, pp. 69–147.

Schneider, J., Section, I.V., 1977. The EEG report. In: Remond, A. (Ed.), Handbook of Electroencephalography and Clinical Neurophysiology, vol. II A. Elsevier, Amsterdam, pp. 97–109.

Appendix 1
Influence of common drugs on the EEG and on seizure threshold

Many common medications have effects on the brain and thus on the EEG. Although these effects are not specific, it is important for our readers to be familiar with them in order to avoid an erroneous diagnosis of intrinsic brain pathology.

ANTI-DEPRESSANTS

Tricyclic anti-depressants such as imipramine, amitriptyline, doxepin, desipramine, and nortriptyline usually increase the amount of beta activity, as well as theta activity in the record. The frequency of the PDR is usually decreased. Paroxysmal slow waves or even spikes may be seen. In patients with epilepsy, seizure frequency could be increased. With high doses, seizures have been reported in patients without a history of epilepsy. Acute intoxication may produce widespread poorly reactive alpha-range activity and spikes. Absence status can be seen with tricyclic anti-depressants.

Of the newer anti-depressants, bupropion stands out as lowering the seizure threshold with a rate of seizures of about 1.5%. There are no definite effects on the EEG of the newer anti-depressants.

Of note, selective serotonin reuptake inhibitors (SSRI) and other anti-depressants can cause serotonin syndrome with mental status changes, autonomic instability, myoclonus, and tremor. The EEG in serotonin syndrome can show diffuse slowing, spikes, and generalized periodic discharges with a triphasic morphology.

With the exception of trazodone, nearly all anti-depressants have been noted to decrease REM sleep with variable effects on stage I, II, and slow wave sleep.

ANTI-EPILEPTIC DRUGS

Phenytoin, unlike barbiturates and benzodiazepines, does not produce prominent beta activity. Rather, it tends to cause an increase in the degree of diffuse slow waves in the theta range. With chronic use there is usually a decline in the frequency of the PDR. At toxic levels, diffuse irregular delta activity may be recorded along with paroxysmal rhythmic delta activity.

Carbamazepine and oxcarbazepine usually have little effect on the EEG at therapeutic levels. An increase in diffuse slowing may occur. Epileptiform activity is usually not materially altered, although an increase in focal spikes has been reported. Rarely, generalized epileptiform potentials develop. Vigabatrin is also associated with the development of generalized epileptiform potentials occasionally with absence of myoclonic seizures.

Valproic acid at therapeutic levels produces little or no change in the EEG background. Its principal effect is a reduction in generalized epileptiform discharges, particularly 3 Hz generalized spike and wave discharges. At toxic levels, valproate may produce an encephalopathy characterized by lethargy with a recording dominated by diffuse delta waves.

Lamotrigine decreases the frequency of interictal spikes and sharp waves and is not associated with either increased beta activity or increased slowing. Lamotrigine can worsen (or ameliorate) myoclonic seizures. Levetiracetam decreases interictal epileptiform potentials typically without other effects on the EEG. Ethosuximide decreases generalized spike and wave and absence seizures.

As of this writing, there are a multitude of other AEDs whose effect on the EEG is either minor and/or not fully investigated.

ANTI-MICROBIAL AGENTS

β-lactam antibiotics, specifically penicillin, the cephalosporins and the carbapenems, are well known to be pro-convulsant, causing an altered mental status, jerks, generalized seizures and even status epilepticus. The β-lactam ring can bind to the GABA receptor making GABA a less effective inhibitory neurotransmitter. For all of these agents, risk factors in the development of seizures include high doses, renal failure, and meningitis. Of all of these agents, imipenum, a carbapenem, is the worst culprit, causing seizures in approximately one third of patients with meningitis. The EEG with β-lactam induced encephalopathy is usually slow with generalized epileptiform potentials, at times with a triphasic morphology. Isoniazid and the flouroquinolones are also known to lower the seizure threshold.

BARBITURATES

Barbiturates produce an increase in the amount and amplitude of beta activity. The beta may reach high amplitudes and, although diffuse, is often most prominent in the frontal regions. As the blood level of the barbiturate rises, slower activity begins to invade the recording along with slowing of the PDR. Barbiturate intoxication leads to changes similar to those associated with general anesthesia. Diffuse, unreactive delta activity may be recorded, while beta activity disappears. Later stages lead to burst-suppression and ultimately an isopotential or flat record. Abrupt withdrawal after long-term treatment may lead to asynchronous slowing along with generalized epileptiform activity.

BENZODIAZEPINES

Like barbiturates, benzodiazepines produce prominent beta activity. Even after the last dose of one of these drugs, excessive beta may persist for some days. Some diffuse theta range slowing may be seen along with attenuation of the PDR. Paroxysmal synchronous slowing may be seen after long-term use. Effects of toxic doses are similar to those produced by other CNS depressants and correlate with degree of mental status depression. Benzodiazepines have been shown to decrease the amount of stage 1 sleep (which can be helpful in people who suffer from insomnia) and decrease slow wave sleep.

CNS TOXINS

There are a great number of agents which are toxic to the CNS and can cause acute, subacute or chronic neurological symptoms. These include but are not limited to toxicity with lead, mercury, methyl alcohol, carbon monoxide and organophosphate poisoning. The EEG findings are not specific for any one culprit and can include diffuse slowing and generalized epileptiform abnormalities. Focal epileptiform discharges have been reported as well.

ETHANOL

Chronic alcoholics often have an EEG which is low in amplitude. In the first 48 hours of alcohol withdrawal syndrome, the EEG may be low in amplitude with generalized spikes or even lateralized periodic discharges (LPDs). Seizures and even status epilepticus are a well known complication of alcohol withdrawal, particularly in the period of 6–48 hours after alcohol cessation. Alcohol withdrawal seizures are treated in the short term, usually with benzodiazepines, but other AEDs, like carbamazepine or topiramate, appear to be effective and safe. If epileptiform features persist after the period of acute withdrawal, the clinician should consider the possibility of non-alcohol related seizures as well. Outside of alcohol withdrawal, chronic alcoholics have a three-fold increased risk of developing epilepsy compared with the general population. While this is not fully understood, increased head trauma, cardiovascular disease, kindling with alcohol withdrawal seizures, and/or general poor nutrition and health are thought to contribute to the overall risk. Patients with epilepsy are advised to minimize alcohol intake, as a seizure can follow even a single night of moderate to heavy drinking.

LITHIUM

Lithium may lead to diverse and prominent changes in the EEG. Although there is some correlation between the blood level of lithium and electrographic changes, there is considerable variability. One may see slowing of the PDR along with an increase in diffuse slowing. Intermittent rhythmic delta waves, most prominent in the frontal or occipital regions, may appear, and triphasic waves have been described. Occasional spikes and focal slowing should not be interpreted as evidence of a structural lesion. With lithium intoxication, EEG abnormalities are usually marked and include considerable diffuse slow waves, triphasic waves, and multifocal epileptiform discharges. These findings may linger for days after clinical manifestations of intoxication have resolved.

MARIJUANA

Smoking marijuana produces no visible changes on EEG. There is a recent surge in interest on the potential of cannabidiol, a compound in marijuana, as a potential AED.

NEUROLEPTICS

Typical neuroleptics (e.g., phenothiazines) at therapeutic doses cause slowing of the PDR along with diffuse slow waves. They may also activate generalized delta activity and sharp waves. In epileptic patients, phenothiazines may increase seizure frequency, particularly at high or toxic doses.

The atypical neuroleptic, clozapine, produces an increase in diffuse slowing. Chronic use may lead to paroxysmal slowing with spikes or sharp waves. More than other neuroleptics, clozapine lowers the seizure threshold and has been reported to cause GTC seizures and myoclonic jerks. Other atypical neuroleptics (olanzapine, quetiapine and risperidone) have very little effect on the EEG.

STIMULANT MEDICATION AND DRUGS

The question of the safety of CNS stimulants in those with epilepsy is not uncommon as attention difficulties and epilepsy can be comorbid. If the epilepsy is well controlled, increased seizures are generally not seen in patients on stimulants. However, in uncontrolled or refractory epilepsy, methylphenidate has been shown to increase seizures. Stimulants can increase the abundance of alpha and beta in the EEG and decrease the overall voltage. Stimulants, not surprisingly, increase the amount of time spent in stage I sleep and have been reported to decrease slow wave and REM sleep. Intoxication with stimulants at high doses can show an abnormal and encephalopathic EEG with diffuse slowing and epileptiform abnormalities. Cocaine increases the amount of beta in the EEG and is well known to lower the seizure threshold in people with epilepsy and in people with no prior history of seizures. Cocaine has been known to cause status epilepticus.

THE ROLE OF THE EEG IN DETERMINING ANTI-EPILEPTIC DRUG TREATMENT

The EEG plays a potentially useful role in selecting an appropriate AED. Although there may be sufficient information to make an informed decision on the basis of the clinical picture, this can be misleading. For example, in cases of GTCC it is not necessarily obvious whether the seizures are primarily or secondarily generalized. Likewise, in patients with apparent absence seizures, the clinical differentiation from complex partial seizures may be difficult. In both these instances the EEG offers assistance.

In individuals with absence seizures, one should select an agent that might be considered as an "anti-spike-wave" AED such as valproate. Topiramate and lamotrigine are also considerations. If the EEG picture and clinical evidence are diagnostic of simple absence epilepsy without concomitant GTCC or myoclonus, ethosuximide is an excellent choice. If the EEG reveals a temporal spike focus in a patient with apparent confusional states, the choice would be one of the "focal" agents, either one of the newer agents (e.g., lacosamide) or one of the older agents such as carbamazepine, oxcarbazepine, gabapentin. If, on the other hand, the EEG is indeterminate (i.e., a decision cannot be made between a focal or generalized abnormality [the EEG might be normal]), then selection of a broad-spectrum agent would be a rational choice (e.g., levetiracetam, lamotrigine, topiramate). Older agents such as phenytoin, valproate, or phenobarbital have a higher side effect profile and are usually not first-line choices. Some of the agents used to treat partial epilepsy, particularly carbamazepine, oxcarbazepine, phenytoin, gabapentin, pregabalin and vigabatrin may make generalized epilepsy worse, particularly absence seizures. It is not yet known if some of the agents recently approved for partial epilepsy like ezogabine and lacosamide are efficacious for generalized onset seizures. However, perampanel is the first agent in over 15 years to be approved for primary generalized tonic-clonic seizures in patients with idiopathic generalized epilepsy.

Further reading

Bauer, G., Bauer, R., 2011. EEG, drug effects and central nervous system poisoning. In: Niedermeyer's Electrencephalography: Basic Principles, Clinical applications, and Related Fields, 6 ed. Lippincott Williams & Wilkins Health, Philadelphia, PA.

Chan, A.W.K., 1985. Alcoholism and epilepsy. Epilepsia 26, 323–333.

Denny-Brown, D.E., Swan, R.L., Foley, I.M., 1947. Respiratory and electrical signs in barbiturate intoxications. Trans. Am. Neurol. Assoc. 77, 77.

Eriksson, A.S., Knutsson, E., Nergardh, A., 2001. The effect of lamotrigine on epileptiform discharges in young patients with drug-resistant epilepsy. Epilepsia 42, 230–236.

Fink, M., 1968. EEG and human psychopharmacology. Annu. Rev. Pharmacol. 9, 241–258.

French, J.A., Krauss, G.L., Wechsler, R.T., 2015. Perampanel for tonic-clonic seizures in idiopathic generalized epilepsy: A randomized trial. Neurology 84 no. 14 Supplement S31.007.

French, J.A., Pedley, T.A., 2008. Clinical practice. Initial management of epilepsy. N Engl J Med 359, 166–176.

Gibbs, F.A., Gibbs, E.L., Lennox, W.G., 1937. Effect on the electroencephalogram of certain drugs which influence nervous activity. Arch. Intern. Med. 60, 154–166.

Gross-Tsur, V., 1997. Epilepsy and attention deficit hyperactivity disorder: is methylphenidate safe and effective? J. Pediatr. 130, 670–674.

Haider, J., Matthew, H., Oswald, J., 1971. Electroencephalographic changes in acute drug poisoning. Electroencephalogr. Clin. Neurophysiol. 30, 23–31.

Harvey, S.C., 1975. Hypnotics and sedatives. The barbiturates. In: Goodman, L.S., Gilman, A. (Eds.), The Pharmacological Basis of Therapeutics. Macmillan, New York, pp. 102–123.

Herkes, G.K., Lagerlund, T.D., Sharbrough, F.W., et al., 1993. Effects of antiepileptic drug treatment on the background frequency of EEGs in epileptic patients. J. Clin. Neurophysiol. 10, 210–216.

Hughes, J.R., 2009. Alcohol withdrawal seizures. Epilepsy Behav. 15 (2), 92–97.

Hollister, L.E., Barthel, C.A., 1959. Changes in the electroencephalogram during chronic administration of the tranquilizing drugs. Electroencephalogr. Clin. Neurophysiol. 11, 792–795.

Kochen, S., Gigante, B., Oddo, S., 2002. Spike-wave complexes and seizure exacerbation caused by carbamazepine. Eur. J. Neurol. 9, 41–47.

Kugler, J., Lorenzi, E., Spatz, R., et al., 1979. Drug-induced paroxysmal EEG activities. Pharmacopsychiatry 12, 165–172.

Kurtz, D., 1976. The EEG in acute and chronic drug intoxications. In: Glaser, G.H. (Ed.), Metabolic and Toxic Diseases/Handbook of Electroencephalography and Clinical Neurophysiology, vol. 15. Elsevier, Amsterdam, pp. 88–104.

Marciani, M.G., Gigli, G.L., Stefanini, F., et al., 1993. Effect of carbamazepine on EEG background activity and on interictal epileptiform abnormalities in focal epilepsy. Int. J. Neurosci. 70, 107–116.

Marciani, M.G., Stanzione, P., Maschio, M., et al., 1997. EEG changes induced by vigabatrin monotherapy in focal epilepsy. Acta Neurol. Scand. 95, 115–120.

Marciani, M.G., Stanzione, P., Mattia, D., et al., 1998. Lamotrigine add-on therapy in focal epilepsy: electroencephalographic and neuropsychological evaluation. Clin. Neuropharmacol. 21, 41–47.

Talwar, D., Arora, M.S., Sher, P.K., 1994. EEG changes and seizure exacerbation in young children treated with carbamazepine. Epilepsia 35, 1154–1159.

Toman, J.E.P., Davis, J.P., 1949. The effects of drugs upon the electrical activity of the brain. J. Pharmacol. Exp. Ther. 97, 425–492.

Van Sweden, B., Dumon-Radermecker, M., 1982. The EEG in chronic psychotropic drug intoxications. Clin. Electroencephalogr. 13, 206–215.

Appendix 2
Treatment of Status Epilepticus

In status epilepticus each case must be individually analyzed. The treatment of epilepsia partialis continua with no impairment in mental status will be far less aggressive than the treatment of convulsive status epilepticus. However, certain tenets remain the same. In every patient who has status epilepticus, the first step is heeding the basics and making sure that airway, breathing, and circulation are secure. If IV access has been achieved, then thiamine and glucose along with an abortive medication (lorazepam 0.1 mg/kg is the best choice) are given simultaneously. If there is no IV access, IM midazolam is an excellent alternative. An underlying cause, particularly causes that are easily reversible (hypoglycemia) or life-threatening (meningitis or an epidural hematoma), are sought with physical examination labs, imaging, and a lumbar puncture if needed.

If seizure activity does not cease, fosphenytoin 20 mg/kg or phenytoin 20 mg/kg IV is given. Fosphenytoin/phenytoin should be avoided in individuals (usually children) who have a known myoclonic form of epilepsy. In this instance, valproate is a reasonable choice in children older than 2 years of age. If seizures do not break with fosphenytoin/ phenytoin, the next step is largely institution/physician dependent, but

intubation and preparation for a continuous infusion are not unreasonable. Choice of other agents to add largely depends on the patient and comorbid conditions. If a patient is acidotic, topiramate would be a poor choice as it can cause a metabolic acidosis. Similarly, valproate is avoided in patients with liver disease because it can be hepatotoxic.

The goal of treatment of status epilepticus is eradication of both electrographic and clinical signs of status epilepticus, as well as appropriate diagnosis and treatment of any underlying condition causing the status epilepticus. Any individual in status epilepticus that clinically remits but who is not back to his or her baseline must be connected to a continuous VEEG as there is often no clinical difference between a post-ictal state and ongoing non-convulsive status epilepticus (NCSE). For individuals who require a continuous infusion to break clinical status, continuous VEEG is necessary because NCSE can persist. While experts may argue on how deep the EEG suppression should be, all would agree that the infusion should suppress all electrographic seizures.

Dosing guidelines for both intermittent medication and continuous infusions for the treatment of status epilepticus follow.

Table Appendix 2-1 Intermittent drug dosing in status epilepticus

Drug	Initial dosing	Administration rates and alternative dosing recommendations	Serious adverse effects	Considerations
Diazepam	0.15 mg/kg IV up to 10 mg per dose, may repeat in 5 min	Up to 5 mg/min (IVP) Peds: 2–5 years, 0.5 mg/kg (PR); 6–11 years, 0.3 mg/kg (PR); older than 12 years, 0.2 mg/kg (PR)	Hypotension Respiratory depression	Rapid redistribution (short duration), active metabolite, IV contains propylene glycol
Lorazepam	0.1 mg/kg IV up to 4 mg per dose, may repeat in 5–10 min	Up to 2 mg/min (IVP)	Hypotension Respiratory depression	Dilute 1:1 with saline IV contains propylene glycol
Midazolam	0.2 mg/kg IM up to maximum of 10 mg	Peds: 10 mg IM (>40 kg); 5 mg IM (13–40 kg); 0.2 mg/kg (intranasal); 0.5 mg/kg (buccal)	Respiratory depression Hypotension	Active metabolite, renal elimination, rapid redistribution (short duration)
Fosphenytoin	20 mg PE/kg IV, may give additional 5 mg/kg	Up to 150 mg PE/min; may give additional dose 10 min after loading infusion Peds: up to 3 mg/kg/min	Hypotension Arrhythmias	Compatible in saline, dextrose, and lactated ringer solutions
Lacosamide	200–400 mg IV	200 mg IV over 15 min No pediatric dosing established	PR prolongation Hypotension	Minimal drug interactions Limited experience in treatment of SE
Levetiracetam	1,000–3,000 mg IV Peds: 20–60 mg/kg IV	2–5 mg/kg/min IV		Minimal drug interactions Not hepatically metabolized
Phenobarbital	20 mg/kg IV, may give an additional 5–10 mg/kg	50–100 mg/min IV, may give additional dose 10 min after loading infusion	Hypotension Respiratory depression	IV contains propylene glycol
Phenytoin	20 mg/kg IV, may give an additional 5–10 mg/kg	Up to 50 mg/min IV; may give additional dose 10 min after loading infusion Peds: up to 1 mg/kg/min	Arrhythmias Hypotension Purple glove syndrome	Only compatible in saline IV contains propylene glycol

Table Appendix 2-1 continued

Drug	Initial dosing	Administration rates and alternative dosing recommendations	Serious adverse effects	Considerations
Topiramate	200–400 mg NG/PO	300–1,600 mg/day orally (divided 2–4 times daily) No pediatric dosing established	Metabolic acidosis	No IV formulation available
Valproate sodium	20–40 mg/kg IV, may give an additional 20 mg/kg	3–6 mg/kg/min, may give additional dose 10 min after loading infusion Peds (older than 2 years): 1.5–3 mg/kg/min	Hyperammonemia Pancreatitis Thrombocytopenia Hepatotoxicity	Use with caution in patients with traumatic head injury; may be a preferred agent in patients with glioblastoma multiforme

IM intramuscular; *IV* intravenous; *IVP* intravenous push; *min* minute; *NG* nasogastric; *PE* phenytoin equivalents; *Peds* pediatric; *PO* by mouth; *PR* rectal administration. Reprinted with permission from Neurocritical Care Society Status Epilepticus Guideline Writing Committee. Guidelines for the evaluation and management of status epilepticus. Neurocritical care. 2012;-08; 17:3–23.

Table Appendix 2-2 Continuous infusion dosing guidelines for refractory status epilepticus

Drug	Initial dose	Continuous infusion dosing recommendations – titrated to EEG	Serious adverse effects	Considerations
Midazolam	0.2 mg/kg; administer at an infusion rate of 2 mg/min	0.05–2 mg/kg/hr CI Breakthrough SE: 0.1–0.2 mg/kg bolus, increase CI rate by 0.05–0.1 mg/kg/hr every 3–4 h	Respiratory depression Hypotension	Tachyphylaxis occurs after prolonged use Active metabolite, renally eliminated, rapid redistribution (short duration), does NOT contain propylene glycol
Pentobarbital	5–15 mg/kg, may give additional 5–10 mg/kg; administer at an infusion rate ≤50 mg/min	0.5–5 mg/kg/h CI Breakthrough SE: 5 mg/kg bolus, increase CI rate by 0.5–1 mg/kg/h every 12 h	Hypotension Respiratory depression Cardiac depression Paralytic ileus At high doses, complete loss of neurological function	Requires mechanical ventilation IV contains propylene glycol

Continued

Table Appendix 2-2 continued

Drug	Initial dose	Continuous infusion dosing recommendations – titrated to EEG	Serious adverse effects	Considerations
Propofol	Start at 20 mcg/kg/min, with 1–2 mg/kg loading dose	30–200 mcg/kg/min CI Use caution when administering high doses (>80 mcg/kg/min) for extended periods of time (i.e., >48 h) Peds: Use caution with doses >65 mcg/kg/min; contraindicated in young children Breakthrough SE: Increase CI rate by 5–10 mcg/kg/min every 5 min or 1 mg/kg bolus plus CI titration	Hypotension (especially with loading dose in critically ill patients) Respiratory depression Cardiac failure Rhabdomyolysis Metabolic acidosis Renal failure (PRIS)	Requires mechanical ventilation Must adjust daily caloric intake (1.1 kcal/mL)
Thiopental	2–7 mg/kg, administer at an infusion rate ≤50 mg/min	0.5–5 mg/kg/h CI Breakthrough SE: 1–2 mg/kg bolus, increase CI rate by 0.5–1 mg/kg/h every 12 h	Hypotension Respiratory depression Cardiac depression	Requires mechanical ventilation Metabolized to pentobarbital

CI continuous infusion; *EEG* electroencephalogram; *h* hour; *IM* intramuscular; *IV* intravenous; *IVP* intravenous push; *min* minute; *PRIS* propofol-related infusion syndrome
Reprinted with permission from Neurocritical Care Society Status Epilepticus Guideline Writing Committee. Guidelines for the evaluation and management of status epilepticus. Neurocritical care. 2012;-08; 17:3–23.

Further reading

Lowenstein, D., Alldredge, B., 1998. Status epilepticus. N. Engl. J. Med. 338, 970–976.

Neurocritical Care Society Status Epilepticus Guideline Writing Committee G, 2012. Guidelines for the evaluation and management of status epilepticus. Neurocrit. Care 17, 3–23.

Silbergleit, R., Lowenstein, D., Durkalski, V., et al. and the Neurological Emergency Treatment Trials (NETT) Investigators, 2011. RAMPART (Rapid Anticonvulsant Medication Prior to Arrival Trial): A double-blind randomized clinical trial of the efficacy of intramuscular midazolam versus intravenous lorazepam in the prehospital treatment of status epilepticus by paramedics. Epilepsia 52, 45–47.

Treiman, D.M., Meyers, P.D., Walton, N.Y., et al., 1998. A comparison of four treatments for generalized convulsive status epilepticus. Veterans Affairs Status Epilepticus Cooperative Study Group. N. Engl. J. Med. 339 (12), 792–798.

Glossary

Activité moyenne. Means "average or medium" and refers to the normal full-term neonatal awake and active sleep background. This activity consists of continuous, low to medium voltage activity predominantly in the theta and delta range with overriding beta.

Active sleep. Seen in the neonatal EEG. Typically the EEG is continuous, and there are rapid eye movements (REM) and irregular respirations.

Alpha. Frequencies in the range of 8 to <13 Hz.

Alpha coma. Infrequently seen after a catastrophic brain injury such as anoxia. The patient is comatose, and the EEG shows alpha range activity in widespread distribution, usually maximal in the frontal regions. There is no reactivity as seen with the PDR. Prognosis is poor.

Alpha variants. Variants of the PDR with harmonically related frequencies. Slow alpha variant is half the alpha frequency; fast alpha variant twice. May coexist with alpha or appear alone. Notched appearance of slow alpha variant gives a clue to its presence.

Amplitude. The voltage of the waveform. Measured in microvolts (μV).

A-P gradient. Anterior-posterior gradient. In a normal awake adult EEG there are faster frequencies that are lower in amplitude anteriorly and a well-formed PDR occipitally.

Asynchrony. The opposite of synchrony – that is, the independent or non-simultaneous occurrence of EEG waves over the two hemispheres.

Attenuation. Reduction of EEG activity. An example is reduction or disappearance of the alpha following eye opening.

Background. The underlying activity of the brain. Focal slow waves, synchronous bifrontal slowing, epileptiform discharges, and seizures are said to interrupt the background.

Band. Refers to a frequency range. For example, alpha lies in the 8–13 Hz frequency band.

Beta. Rhythmic, usually low-voltage activity at 13–30 Hz. Usually maximal over the frontocentral regions. Increases in amplitude and becomes more widespread with certain drugs (e.g., benzodiazepines, barbiturates).

BETS. Benign epileptiform transients of sleep. See SSS.

Bilateral synchrony. Refers to waveforms appearing simultaneously over both hemispheres, often applied to generalized spike-wave complexes (e.g., as seen in simple absence attacks). A focal discharge can have secondary rapid bilateral synchrony and be indistinguishable on surface electrodes from a generalized discharge.

Bipolar recording. Recording that compares the activity at two neighboring electrodes with one electrode in Input 1 and the second electrode in Input 2 of the amplifier. The phase reversal is the localization principle of bipolar recording.

BIRDs. Brief potentially ictal rhythmic discharges (BIRDs). Very brief (<10 seconds, typically 0.5–4 seconds) runs of focal or generalized rhythmic activity greater than 4 Hz without evolution. They are associated with high risk of seizures and are highly correlated with the seizure focus.

GLOSSARY

Breach rhythm. Term referring to localized increased amplitude of background rhythms that result from an underlying craniotomy or break in the calvarium (Breach: a broken or torn place. *Webster's World College Dictionary*, 4th ed.) Beta activity with admixed slower frequencies may appear quite sharp and should not be mistaken for epileptiform discharges.

Burst suppression. Episodic or paroxysmal potentials, slow or sharp, or a combination of both, followed by suppression of cerebral activity. Suppressions vary widely in duration.

CA. Conceptual age is the sum of the gestational age (the number of weeks since the last menstrual cycle) and the legal age (age since time of birth).

Channel. Refers to the output of an amplifier that displays electrical information. The number of channels displayed by an EEG apparatus varies.

Common average reference recording. Referential montage in which the activity from the exploring electrode is compared with the averaged activity of the remaining electrodes on the scalp.

Common mode rejection. A signal that is the same in the two amplifier inputs is "rejected" and not displayed, as there is no potential difference.

Common mode signal. Any activity, either physiological or environmental, that is the same at the two inputs of an amplifier.

Complex. The pattern of two or more distinct wave forms. The best example is the spike-wave complex in which each discharge has the same temporal relationship of the spike to the following wave.

Delta. Frequencies in the 0.5 to <4 Hz frequency band.

Delta brush. A slow, moderate- to high-amplitude delta wave with superimposed lower-amplitude fast frequencies. Common in the neonatal EEG. Also sometimes seen in EEGs in persons with NMDA limbic encephalitis.

Depression. Refers to reduction of amplitude or voltage due to a disease process, focal or generalized. An example would be the depression of amplitude sometimes recorded over a subdural hematoma or hygroma.

Derivation. Recording from an electrode pair with the output displayed in one channel of the recording.

Differential amplifier. An amplifier whose output is proportional to the difference in voltage between the two input terminals.

Diffuse. Occurring generally over the two hemispheres, usually used to describe slowing. Contrast with focal slowing.

Discharge. Used to describe a paroxysmal event (e.g., a spike), or electrographic ictal activity (e.g., a new paroxysmal rhythmic frequency).

Electrode impedance. Opposition to AC current flow between an electrode and its interface with the scalp. Measured between pairs of electrodes and measured in Ohms (thousands of Ohms in EEG work). It is important that electrode impedances are generally equal and relatively low in order to ensure good, artifact-free recording.

Electrographic seizure. Recorded ictal activity with or without clinical accompaniment. May be focal with recruiting rhythms or generalized.

Encoches frontales. Frontal sharp waves in the neonatal period, which may occur in isolation or in brief runs.

EPC. Epilepsia partialis continua. Ongoing focal clonic motor seizures without impairment of consciousness. Often does not have an electrographic correlate.

Epileptiform discharges. Refers to polyspikes, spikes, spike-wave complexes, and sharp waves.

Equipotential. Term used to indicate equal potentials at different electrodes.

Exploring electrode. The designation of an electrode that records cerebral activity of interest.

Fast activity. Synonym for beta or gamma activity.

Focus. Refers to the location of maximal potential, usually electronegative.

Fourteen and six positive spikes (14/6). Electropositive spikes at 14 or 6 Hz, or a combination of both. Usually maximal in the posterior temporal derivations and best recorded with wide interelectrode distances (e.g., the crossed ear reference). Of doubtful clinical significance.

Frontally predominant GRDA (aka FIRDA – frontal intermittent rhythmic delta activity). High-voltage bifrontal rhythmic waves, which are non-specific but may be indicative of increased intracranial pressure, deep structural lesions, toxic metabolic states, or other encephalopathies. If this activity appears during sleep onset in the elderly it is considered normal.

Half alpha variant. Normal variant seen in children after age 8. One-half the frequency of the PDR. Notched appearance.

High-frequency filter (aka low pass filter). Attenuates high frequencies (passes all the low frequencies, filters out high frequencies). Can be adjusted by a stepped control available on all EEG machines and digital reading stations.

Hyperventilation. Standard procedure during routine EEG recording. The subject is asked to overbreathe deeply at a faster than normal rate for a period of 3–5 minutes. Often activates latent abnormalities, especially the generalized spike-wave discharges seen in childhood absence epilepsy.

Hypnogogic hypersynchrony. Diffuse semi-rhythmic high voltage slow waves lasting for several seconds in drowsiness. Seen in children older than 6 months of age.

Hypnopompic hypersynchrony. Diffuse semi-rhythmic high-voltage slow waves lasting for several seconds upon arousal. Seen in children older than 6 months of age.

Hypsarrhythmia. Chaotic, very high-voltage discharges consisting of an admixture of generalized spikes, sharp waves, and slow waves, characteristic of West syndrome. One may also see focal discharges, as well as intermittent suppression of cerebral activity.

Input I. Refers to the first of two inputs to an amplifier (Lead 1).

Input II. Refers to the second of two inputs to an amplifier (Lead 2).

Interelectrode distance. Distance between pairs of electrodes.

Isolated. Refers to a waveform (e.g., a spike or slow wave) occurring as an individual, non-repetitive event.

Isopotentiality. Term used for lack of electrocortical potentials. Seen after severe cerebral damage secondary to cardiopulmonary arrest or during deep anesthesia. Sometimes referred to as "flat line".

K-complexes. High-voltage mono- or multiphasic paroxysmal slow potentials often found with sleep spindles. Prominent during stage II sleep. May be triggered during sleep by a loud sound (**K**nock) with no clinical signs of arousal or transition out of sleep.

Lambda waves. Electropositive sharp potentials recorded in the occipital regions (like an evoked potential), generated when a subject is visually scanning the environment (often while reading).

Lead. Refers to an electrode and its connection to the EEG machine.

Low-frequency filter (aka high-pass filter). Attenuates low frequencies (passes all the high frequencies, filters out all the low frequencies). Can be adjusted by a stepped control available on all EEG machines and digital reading stations.

Montage. Term used to indicate the arrangement of electrodes displaying the EEG activity.

Monorhythmic occipital delta. Runs of high amplitude posterior delta. Seen in premature neonates.

Multifocal sharp transients. Sharp waves seen throughout the EEG in normal neonates.

Nasopharyngeal electrode. Relatively thin, insulated wire with an exposed tip, introduced through the nose, coming to rest as the back of the nasopharynx adjacent to the sphenoid bone. Records activity from the inferior temporal or frontal lobe. Used less frequently today secondary to discomfort and artifact (e.g., respiratory, swallowing, pulse).

Noise. Small currents in an EEG channel related to the machine circuitry, not physiological potentials.

Notch filter. A circuit that filters out a narrow band of frequencies (e.g., a 60 Hz notch filter [50 Hz in UK]) removes the most common electrical artifact. Particularly important when recording in ICU settings, where a variety of electrical equipment is in use.

Mu rhythm. Mu rhythm is a normal finding. It appears as sharply contoured rhythmic waves at 7–11 Hz, maximal over the central regions. May be unilateral or bilateral. Attenuates with movement of the opposite upper extremity (e.g., making a fist) or even thinking about moving the contralateral arm.

Organization. A well-organized adult waking EEG usually contains PDR in the occipital regions, beta activity in the frontocentral regions, and little else. If the PDR is disrupted by slower frequencies, the record might be said to be somewhat disorganized with intermittent generalized slowing. If there is no PDR along with a great deal of generalized delta range slowing, the record might be said to be disorganized and slow.

Parodoxical alpha. Alpha rhythm that appears after eye opening, seen in drowsy subjects (the opposite of what happens in alert subjects).

Paroxysm. Term used to indicate a waveform that arises suddenly from the background (e.g., a spike discharge).

PDR. Posterior dominant rhythm. In the alpha frequency (8 to <13 Hz) in the posterior regions of the head. The PDR attenuates with eye opening and is best seen when the person is in the relaxed, waking state with eyes closed.

193

PDs. Periodic discharges (aka PEDs, or periodic epileptiform discharges). Can be generalized (GPDs) as is often seen post cardiac arrest or lateralized (LPDs) adjacent to an area of cerebral infarction or tumor. These discharges are not always spikes (hence elimination of the "E") but are typically epileptiform nonetheless.

Periodicity. Refers to recurrent focal or generalized discharges with a relatively fixed interdischarge interval (the period).

Phantom spike-wave. A normal variant characterized by low-voltage 6 Hz spike wave discharges.

Phase reversal. Localization principle of bipolar recording. The electrical phenomenon of interest (e.g., a sharp wave or spike) point toward each other in adjacent channels.

Photic driving. Response to intermittent photic stimulation recorded in the occipital regions. The evoked waves are time-locked to the flash rate. If there is a 1:1 response, it is termed *the fundamental*. If the response is twice the flash frequency, it is termed *a harmonic response*, and if half the frequency it is termed *the subharmonic*. All are normal.

Photomyoclonic response. Response to intermittent photic stimulation consisting of repetitive muscle action potentials, maximal in the frontal derivations, linked to the flash frequency. A normal response that ceases when the flash train stops.

Photoparoxysmal response (aka photoconvulsive response). Generalized, synchronous epileptiform activity consisting of spike and polyspike wave complexes, maximal in the frontal regions, evoked by intermittent photic stimulation. When recorded, the technician must stop the flash stimulus immediately to avoid the possibility of precipitating a generalized seizure. The response usually outlasts cessation of the flash train by 1–2 seconds. The response is not always convulsive in nature.

Photosensitivity. General term in denoting an abnormal response to intermittent photic stimulation including the photoparoxysmal response. With lesser degrees of photosensitivity, occipital spikes or generalized spikes or sharp waves are time-locked to the flash frequency. The response stops when the flash train ceases.

PNEA. Psychogenic non-epileptic attacks. A seizure mimic thought to be a conversion or somatiform disorder.

POSTs (aka lambdoidal waves). Positive occipital sharp transients of sleep. Electropositive sharp potentials (in a referential recording), maximal in the occipital derivations. May be quite prominent. Often noted during Stage II sleep. May occur in rhythmic runs.

Posterior slow waves of youth. Occur commonly between 2 and 21 years of age. In the delta range, consisting of 3–6 fused alpha waves. Attenuates with eye opening like the PDR.

Quiet sleep. In the newborn. Respirations are regular and the EEG can show a tracé discontinu, tracé alternant, or continuous pattern.

RDA. Rhythmic Delta Activity. Can be lateralized (LRDA) or generalized (GRDA). If this activity occurs in the temporal region (TRDA), it can be indicative of temporal lobe epilepsy. If occipital (ORDA), it can be indicative of absence epilepsy.

Reactivity. Alteration of EEG activity by external sensory stimulation. In a comatose patient, this is a favorable sign.

Reference recording. Electrodes in input 1 and 2 are not immediately adjacent on the scalp. In referential recording the activity from an exploring electrode (input 1) is compared with the reference, which is out of the field of interest, e.g., the ear (A1/A2) or vertex (Cz) (input 2). In referential recording, the localization principle is amplitude.

REM sleep. Rapid eye movement sleep. Stage of sleep characterized by rapid eye movements, loss of muscle tone, and yes, dreams.

RMTD. Rhythmic midtemporal theta aka psychomotor variant. Normal variant. Rhythmic 4–7 Hz waves in the temporal regions, recorded during drowsiness. May be notched in appearance.

Sensitivity. Ratio of input voltage to output recorded in a channel of the EEG recording.

Sharp-slow complex. Epileptiform pattern consisting of a sharp wave followed by a slow wave, usually in the delta frequency band. A typical example is the generalized sharp-slow complex at 2 Hz, typical of the Lennox–Gastaut syndrome.

Sharp wave. Paroxysmal sharp potential with duration of 70–200 ms. These are longer in duration than spikes but with very similar significance.

Sleep spindles. Rhythmic, sometimes spindle-shaped activity at 12 to 14 Hz (±2), indicative of stage II sleep. Usually maximal over the central region. These waves are mediated by cells in the nucleus reticularis of the thalamus.

Slowing. Brain waves that oscillate at a slower frequency than what would be expected for a particular region. Can be focal or generalized. Can be monomorphic or polymorphic.

Sphenoidal electrodes. Insulated electrode wires with an exposed tip, introduced through the mandibular notch via a hollow needle. After the needle comes to rest near the foramen ovale, the needle is withdrawn. Records activity from the anterior tip of the temporal lobe.

Spike. Paroxysmal potential with duration of 20–70 msec. More rapid rise than fall time; often followed by low-voltage slow potential.

Spike-wave complex. Spike followed by time-locked, high-voltage slow wave. Various frequency bands (typically 3–5 Hz). Synchronous, rhythmic 3 Hz spike-wave runs are typical of simple absence attacks. Synchronous 4–5 Hz spike-wave runs are seen in primary generalized epilepsy with generalized convulsions. Irregular rapid spike-wave discharges are typical of juvenile myoclonic epilepsy (JME).

Spread. Activity spreading out from its site of origin (e.g., PDR that is represented anterior to the occipital regions).

SREDA. Subclinical rhythmic electroencephalographic discharges of adults. A normal variant. Can be mistaken for focal electrographic seizure activity.

SSS. Small sharp spikes aka BETS (benign epileptiform transients of sleep). Low-amplitude, rapid spikes. They appear in both hemispheres as synchronous or asynchronous, most often in the temporal derivations, and become evident during drowsiness and light sleep. Normal variant.

SWS. Slow wave sleep. Predominantly delta activity.

Symmetry. Amplitude comparison between right and left hemispheres.

Synchrony. Waveforms that are spatially independent (e.g., occipital, frontal) occur simultaneously and have a constant phase relationship.

Temporal sawtooth. Sharply contoured rhythmic theta in the temporal electrodes. Seen between 26 and 32 weeks CA.

Theta. Waves in the 4 to <8 Hz frequency band. May be a normal finding or may indicate pathology. Some theta is acceptable in the normal waking adult EEG.

Tracé alternant. Normal pattern found in newborns during quiet sleep characterized by bursts of continuous activity alternating with periods of lower voltage. In tracé alternant, the interburst interval is shorter than in tracé discontinu and slightly higher in amplitude.

Tracé discontinu. The normal discontinuous tracing encountered in healthy preterm babies, which consists of bursts of high-voltage activity interrupted by low-voltage interburst periods.

Triphasic waves. Paroxysmal potentials associated with hepatic encephalopathy or other metabolic encephalopathies. Quite sharp in configuration with three phases, synchronous, maximal bifrontally. Can have an anterior to posterior lag with the first deflection happening slightly sooner anteriorly than posteriorly.

Vertex sharp waves. Recorded during stage II sleep but also noted during late drowsiness. May be high voltage, isolated or repetitive and can be as sharp as spikes. Usually maximal in the central regions (C3, C4, Cz).

Wicket spikes. Sharply contoured rhythmic frequencies varying from 7–11 Hz, maximal in the midtemporal derivations, occurring in brief runs. Normal variant.

Index